A.

Ox

New Trends in Osteoarthritis

Rheumatology

An Annual Review

Vol. 7

Series Editor
M. Schattenkirchner, München

S. Karger · Basel · München · Paris · London · New York · Sydney

New Trends in Osteoarthritis

Volume Editors
E.C. Huskisson, London
G. Katona, Mexico

87 figures, 1 color plate and 75 tables, 1982

S. Karger · Basel · München · Paris · London · New York · Sydney

Rheumatology
An Annual Review

Contents

Tiaprofenic Acid: Clinical Trials

Introduction

Osteoarthritis is a very common and important disease. It is also a disease to which the attitudes of those involved with it have changed in recent years. These changes were discussed and updated when a group of interested physicians, surgeons and scientists met in Monte Carlo in October 1981. They looked at the facts of the disease, its epidemiology, clinical and pathological features and tried to see how chemical and mechanical approaches to the happenings in cartilage might explain them. Treatment was reviewed in the light of new ideas such as the importance of inflammation and the profile of a new nonsteroidal anti-inflammatory drug was presented. This volume is the outcome of the discussions which took place.

E.C. Huskisson
G. Katona

Rheumatology, vol. 7, pp. 1–10 (Karger, Basel 1982)

Clinical Features, Diagnostic Criteria, Functional Assessments and Radiological Classifications of Osteoarthritis (Excluding the Spine)

M. Lequesne

Department of Rheumatology, Hôpital Léopold-Bellan, Paris, France

Introduction

During the Renaissance, dermatology was in the hands of barber-surgeons. Until 1930–1940, diseases of the stomach were seen mainly be surgeons, even from the point of view of diagnosis. We can now appreciate how much non surgical specialists, gastro-enterologists, have contributed to the diagnosis and the treatment of patients whose disease has not reached the point where surgery becomes necessary. This is a good example for osteoarthritis (OA) to follow. It would be regrettable to see OA treated by surgeons from its very beginning, which is currently the case in the USA. In France, OA patients are seen first by the rheumatologist, and many advances could be accomplished in the knowledge of OA as a result of a close co-operation between radiologists, rheumatologists, orthopaedic surgeons and pathologists. In fact, OA is the type of disease that needs a multidisciplinary approach, which now includes epidemiological studies.

Except in a few cases, OA of the extremities does not seem to be a generalised disease. Indeed, it is more often localised or shows little, generally articular disease (like Paget's disease of the bones, which involves several osseous areas without an apparent pattern). In fact, as *Solomon* et al. [14] said: 'The term OA could be applied to a range of disorders; it is unhelpful to lump them together.' What *common* features are there between OA of the shoulder, resulting from a rotator cuff tear, OA of the fingers, usually 'primary', and OA of the hip, which in half the cases, originates from a congenital or acquired malformation? These common features only appear at a late stage of the disease.

Some General Considerations

Despite these difficulties due to the polymorphic nature of the disease, it may be useful to consider several highlights of what is known about OA, especially in its primary form.

(1) Nobody knows why primary OA does not occur in the ankle joint or the wrist and rarely in the elbow and metacarpophalangeal joints. Recently, *Cassou* et al. [1] failed to find any real OA of the ankle in a survey of 110 subjects whose ages ranged from 70 to 100 years (mean 79.5 years).

(2) The joints most commonly involved in primary OA are the following: first carpometacarpal; distal interphalangeal and proximal interphalangeal (Heberden's and Bouchard's nodes); hip (about 40% of OA of the hip is primary); knee, and first metatarsophalangeal.

(3) The association between these different types were studied with markedly conflicting results. Regarding OA of the hip and fingers: no significant correlation was found by *Kellgren* et al. [quoted in ref. 16, p. 193] *Yazici* et al. [18], whereas a significant correlation was found by *Roh* [quoted in ref. 14, p. 48], *Stewart* et al. [16] and by *Solomon* et al. [14], but the latter only in males.

(4) Especially in the Anglo-Saxon literature, the inflammatory component of OA is sometimes emphasised [3, 5, 6], but even when the authors point out that the hydroxyapatite crystals found in some OA joints may explain the inflammatory component, they do not dare to assert that it represents the beginning of OA.

There is much evidence against OA being an inflammatory condition, the most striking being the cellular content of the synovial fluid: in a recent study, *Lemaire* et al. [7] found that in 82 OA synovial fluid samples, 81 (98.7%) contained less than 2,000 cells, with a mean of 30% of polymorphonuclears (PMN) whereas in 124 rheumatoid arthritis synovial fluid samples, 116 (94.4%) contained more than 2,000 cells, with a mean 67% of PMN.

In the very well-documented study by *McCarthy* et al. [12] on 'Milwaukee shoulder', OA of the shoulder resulting from a rotator cuff tear, no inflammation was found in the synovial fluid (about 200–300 cells per cubic millimetre, no α_2-macroglobulin) although numerous hydroxyapatite crystals were present. *Dieppe* [2] studied 100 OA patients and compared them with 100 patients with chondrocalcinosis, 26 with hydroxyapatite crystals in their synovial fluid. He concluded that, (a) the presence of hydroxyapatite crystals does not clearly delineate a separate disease entity. Perhaps it only enhances the severity of OA. (b) There is no significant correlation between the presence of crystals and the severity of the inflammatory component in OA.

(5) The definition of OA is one the most difficult points. The area of OA is not the same for the pathologist, the radiologist, the epidemiologist and the clinician despite some overlap between the different fields.

(a) One example from the point of view of the pathologist: as a result of the autopsy on 66 subjects (40 males, mean age 70, and 26 females, mean age 76) *Stankovic* et al. [15] conclude that anatomical OA is much more frequent than 'OA disease', since femoropatellar OA was found in approximately two thirds, including one third with patellar dysplasia and 12.7% with chondrocalcinosis, and femorotibial OA was observed in 55% of the males (17% severe) and 69% of the females (38% with chondrocalcinosis).

(b) Another example from the point of view of the epidemiologist and the clinician: in a remarkable study in 3,091 men and 3,493 women, *Walkenburg* [17] pointed out that more than 50% of the subjects with radiological evidence of degenerative disease have no clinical symptoms. Among this population only 15% of men and 26% of women had consulted their doctors because of rheumatological complaints.

On the other hand there are many 'false positives', i.e. patients with complaints or even physical signs of possible OA in whom X-ray examination did not show any degenerative changes. These vary between 27 and 78%, depending upon the joint considered. Whether these are 'psychosomatic' or 'pre-radiological' OA patients is discussed in that study.

(c) In our experience [9, 11] in an elderly population (from 65 years onwards) attending the hospital as out-patients for non-rheumatological complaints, the prevalence of painless OA of the hip is of the order of 10–12%. According to *Glimet* et al., [4], it is around 14–18% in the knee joint (in most cases femoropatellar).

Diagnostic Criteria and Functional Indices

Osteoarthritis of the Hip
The diagnostic criteria (table I) we proposed for identifying true OA of the hip in a given drug trial [10] obviously involve the condition 'painful hip'. This condition may be excluded in some cases by making a simple clinical or epidemiological check. Some of the points in the table of criteria and exclusions deserve a brief comment:
C2 – In early OA, narrowing of the joint space is sometimes only evident

Table I. Criteria for definite diagnosis of OA of the hip joint

Clinical criteria

C1 At least three of the seven following movements must be limited and painful: flexion, flexion with adduction, extension, external and internal rotation abduction, adduction

Radiological criteria

C2 Narrowing of the acetabulofemoral space in frontal and/or oblique view in standing position

C3 Osteophytes and/or subchondral osteocondensation and/or cyst

Exclusions

1. Avascular necrosis of the femoral head
2. Arthropathy of the hip associated with Paget's disease of ilium or femoral head
3. Chondrocalcinosis
4. Ochronosis
5. Haemochromatosis
6. Haemophilic arthropathy
    } of the hip joint
7. Inflammatory arthritis of the hip (from rheumatoid arthritis, ankylosing spondylitis, psoriatic arthropathy or arthritis of unknown origin) either with or without any other joint involvement
8. Slow infectious arthritis of the hip, especially tuberculous arthritis.
9. Charcot's hip joint
10. Villonodular synovitis
11. Synovial chondromatosis

The three criteria C1, C2 and C3 must be present. All the exclusions must be systematically considered.

Table II. Incidence of the main causes of OA of the hip in 200 consecutive cases [8]

	Incidence, %
Congenital subluxation and dysplasia of the hip	29
Sequela of slipped femoral epiphysis (coxa vara, tilt deformity)	14
Congenital acetabular protrusion	5
Trauma	5
Sports at a high level (football, rugby, judo, tennis)	2
Postural defects (contralateral ankylosis, important shortening of the contralateral lower limb)	1.5
Miscellaneous	5.5
Primary OA of the hip	38

Table III. Functional index for hip OA (FIH)

	Points
Pain	
Nocturnal pain	
Only on movement or in certain attitudes	1
Even without moving	2
Morning stiffness or pain after getting up	
Less than 15 min	1
15 min or more	2
In the standing position for 30 min – resulting in more pain	1
When walking, is the pain occurring	
Only after a certain distance	1
Or from the beginning and increasing	2
Pain or discomfort in sitting position (over extended period)	1
Maximum distance walked	
More than 1 km, but limited	1
About 1 km (about 15 min)	2
From 500 to 900 m (about 8–15 min)	3
From 300 to 500 m	4
From 100 to 300 m	5
Less than 100 m	6
With one walking stick or crutch	+1
With two walking sticks or crutches	+2
Some difficulties in daily life	
Can you put on the socks from the front?	0–2
Can you pick up an object from the floor?	0–2
Can you ascend a flight of stairs?	0–2
Can you enter or leave a car?	0–2
Sexual disability from hip origin	0–2

Answer rating: easily = 0; with difficulty = 1 (or 0.5 or 1.5); impossible = 2.

in the oblique view [8] and not in the frontal view (even in the standing position) especially in cases of either anterosuperior or posterior narrowing of the space.

C3 – In some cases, OA of the hip, especially when it begins at an advanced age, involves only one radiological sign, i.e. narrowing of the space without any bony reaction, no osteophytes, osteocondensation or cysts. But, to accept such a case as an OA, it would be necessary to leave aside the third criteria C3. Therefore, the diagnosis gains in sensitivity but loses too much in specificity. This is a common problem in methodology when making such a decision. The reverse is also true, i.e. hip radiology revealing only a bony reaction without apparent narrowing of the joint space.

The aetiological diagnosis is most important in the presence of OA of the hip. Table II lists the principal causes we found in a series of 200 cases of OA of the hip. These have to be looked for systematically in each case.

After positive, differential and aetiological diagnoses, the last step in the examination is the appraisal of the level of disability. This can be achieved by using the *functional index for hip disease* (FIH) that we proposed in 1979–1981 [10, 11] (table III.) The FIH involves a theoretical maximum of 26 points. The disability may be graded as follows: 14 points = extremely severe; 11–13 points = very severe; 8–10 points = severe; 4–7 points = moderate; 1–3 points = mild.

The FIH is of great significance when deciding on a hip arthroplasty, either a total prosthesis or a double cup, which is justified when the score reaches 10–12 points. It has been shown to be easily reproducible. It was assessed in a double-blind study including 18 patients. The mean deviation was 0.55 points with a maximum of 2 points. The test for a small matched paired series did not show any significant differences ($t = 1.95$; $p < 0.05$).

Furthermore, the FIH and the value of other criteria used to distinguish the placebo period from the indomethacin period were tested in a double-blind cross-over trial (7 days on each treatment) and appeared very good ($p < 0.001$). The statistical significances of assessment criteria were as follows [11]:

1. FIH	$p < 0.001$
2. Investigator's overall opinion	$p < 0.001$
3. Pain level (visual analogue scale)	$p < 0.01$
4. Patient's overall opinion	$p < 0.01$
5. Walking time (25 m)	$p < 0.05$
6. Abduction, flexion	statistically non-significant

As we can see, the subjective or semi-subjective criteria are best. However, the limitations of mobility merit consideration if the aim of the study is to follow the patient in the long term. In practice, the first four criteria can be used by the rheumatologist to appraise the patient once or twice a year and to assess the efficacy of a given drug in a short-term trial. It requires 3–4 min to carry out the FIH and 1–2 min for the other criteria.

Table IV. Criteria for definite diagnostic of OA of the knee

Clinical criteria
C1 Limitation of motion and/or tenderness at the extremes of knee extension or flexion

X-ray criteria (3 films minimum: frontal in standing position; lateral and axial views)
C2 Narrowing of the femorotibial or femoropatellar space
C3 Osteophytes and/or subchondral osteocondensation and/or cyst

Exclusions
 1. Necrosis of the femoral condyle
 2. Arthropathy of the knee associated with juxta-articular Paget's disease of the femur or tibia
 3. Chondrocalcinosis
 4. Haemochromatosis
 5. Ochronosis
 6. Haemophilic arthropathy
 7. Inflammatory arthritis of the knee (from rheumatoid arthritis, ankylosing spondylitis, psoriatic, arthropathy or arthritis of unknown origin) either with or without any other joint involvement
 8. Slow infectious arthropathy of the knee; especially tuberculosis
 9. Charcot's knee joint
10. Villonodular synovitis
11. Synovial chondromatosis

The three criteria C1, C2 and C3 must be present. All the exclusions must be systematically considered.

Osteoarthritis of the Knee

The diagnostic criteria for OA of the knee are similar to those used for the hip joint (table IV) and the exclusions are the same. The proposed functional index for OA of the knee is shown in table V. It is valid for both femoropatellar and femorotibial OA. This index has not yet been statistically evaluated.

Radiological Stage

It is also useful to have an index of the radiological stage of OA. Table VI summarises the different degrees proposed. X-rays are reliable if taken in a *standing position* for OA of the hip (frontal and oblique view), knee (frontal view) and the ankle.

Table V. Functional index for knee OA

	Points
Pain	
Nocturnal pain	
Only on movement or in certain attitudes	1
Even without moving	2
Morning stiffness or pain after getting up	
Less than 15 min	1
15 min or more	2
Is the standing position during 30 min – resulting in more pain	1
When walking, does the pain occur	
Only after certain distance	1
Or from the beginning and does it increase	2
Pain or discomfort when getting up from a seat	1
Maximum distance walked	
More than 1 km, but limited	1
About 1 km (about 15 min)	2
From 500 to 900 m (about 8–15 min)	3
From 300 to 500 m	4
From 100 to 300 m	5
Less than 100 m	6
With one walking stick or crutch	+1
With two walking sticks or crutches	+2
Some difficulties in daily life	
Can you ascend a flight of stairs?	0–2
Can you go down a flight of stairs?	0–2
Can you arrange something on a low shelf while squatting or being on your knees?	0–2
Can you walk on unequal ground?	0–2
Are you suffering from shooting pains and/or sudden lack of support	
in the involved limb?	
Sometimes	1
Often	2

Answer rating: as in the functional index for hip OA

Osteophytes or osteocondensation, without narrowing of the space sometimes reflect OA and sometimes they are a simple sign of ageing in elderly patients. This is the reason why the radiological index proposed is based on narrowing of the space. This index is valid not for diagnosis but only for specifying the stage in a given case of OA already recognised by the diagnostic criteria.

Table VI. Grading of OA of the extremities – Radiological index

Grade

Narrowing of the space
 1 Less than 50%
 2 50%–90%
 3 (almost) complete obliteration

Attrition of bone
 4 Slight 1–3 mm
 5 Marked 4–6 mm
 6 Severe ≥7 mm
+1 *Massive disproportionate osteophytosis*

The X-ray film must be taken in the standing position (lower extremity) or in contraction (upper extremity). For the evaluation of long-term therapeutic trials, the loss of space (narrowing) and of bone (attrition) must be measured in millimetres (even, if possible, half millimetres).

References

1 Cassou, B.; Camus, J.P.; Peyron, J.G.; Delporte, M.P.; Memin, Y.; Affre, J.: Recherche d'une arthrose primitive de la cheville chez les sujets de plus de 70 ans; in Peyron, Epidemiology of osteoarthritis, pp. 180–184 (Ciba-Geigy, Paris 1981).

2 Dieppe, P.: Calcium phosphate crystal deposition and clinical subsets of osteoarthritis; in Peyron, Epidemiology of osteoarthritis, pp. 71–79 (Ciba-Geigy, Paris 1981).

3 Ehrlich, G.E.: Osteoarthritis beginning with inflammation. J. Am. med. Ass. *232:* 157–175 (1975).

4 Glimet, T.; Massé, J.P.; Ryckewaert, A.: Fréquence de la gonarthrose indolore dans une population de 50 femmes et de 50 hommes âgés de plus de 65 ans; in Peyron, Epidemiology of osteoarthritis, pp. 220–223 (Ciba-Geigy, Paris 1981).

5 Huskisson, E.C.: The clinical features of osteoarthritis. Evidence for inflammation and crystal deposition; in Peyron, Epidemiology of osteoarthritis, pp. 62–70 (Ciba-Geigy, Paris 1981).

6 Huskisson, E.C.; Dieppe, P.A.; Tucker, A.; Cannell, L.: Another look at osteoarthritis. Ann. rheum. Dis. *38:* 423–428 (1979).

7 Lemaire, V.; Peltier, A.; Jouvent, C.; Ryckewaert, A.: Résultats de l'examen cytologique du liquide synovial dans diverses arthropathies. Revue Rhum. Mal. ostéo-artic. *48:* 229–234 (1981).

8 Lequesne, M.: Diseases of hip in adult life (Geigy, Paris 1967).

9 Lequesne, M.: La coxarthrose. Critères de diagnostic. Etiologie sur 200 cas. Rôle de la dysplasie congénitale; in Peyron, Epidemiology of osteoarthritis, pp. 198–210 (Ciba-Geigy, Paris 1981).

10 Lequesne, M.; Mery, C.: European guidelines for clinical trials of new antirheumatic drugs. Eular Bull. *9:* 171–175 (1980).

11   Lequesne, M.; Samson, M.: A functional index for hip diseases. Reproducibility. Value
      for discriminating drug's efficacy (Abstract). 5th Int. Congr. Rheum., pp. 778–779 (Expan-
      sion scientifique française, Paris 1981).
12   McCarthy, D.J.; Halverson, P.B.; Carrega, G.F.; Brewer, B.J.; Kozin, F.: 'Milwaukee
      shoulder' – Association of microspheroids containing hydroxyapatite crystals, active colla-
      genase and neutral protease with rotator cuff defects. Arthritis Rheum. *24:* 464–483 (1981).
13   Peyron, J.G.: Epidemiology of osteoarthritis (Ciba-Geigy, Paris 1981).
14   Solomon, L.; Schnitzler, C.; Browett, J.: Osteoarthritis of the hip. The patient behind the
      disease: in Peyron, Epidemiology of osteoarthritis, pp. 40–52 (Ciba-Geigy, Paris 1981).
15   Stankovic, A.; Mitrouic, D.; Ryckewaert, A.: Prevalence of the degenerative lesions in ar-
      ticular cartilage of the human knee joint. Relationship with age; in Peyron, Epidemiology
      of osteoarthritis, pp. 94–98 (Ciba-Geigy, Paris 1981).
16   Stewart, I.M.; Marks, J.S.; Hardinge, K.: Generalised osteoarthrosis and hip disease; in
      Peyron, Epidemiology of osteoarthritis, pp. 193–197 (Ciba-Geigy, Paris 1981).
17   Walkenburg, H.A.: Clinical versus radiological osteoarthrosis in the general population;
      in Peyron, Epidemiology of osteoarthritis, pp. 53–55 (Ciba-Geigy, Paris 1981).
18   Yazici; Saville, P.D.; Salvati, E.A.; Bohne, W.H.O.; Wilson, P.D.: Primary osteoarthritis
      of the knee or hip. Prevalence of Heberden's nodes in relation to age and sex. J. Am. med.
      Ass. *231:* 1256–1260 (1975).

M. Lequesne, MD, Department of Rheumatology, Hôpital Léopold-Bellan,
F-75116 Paris (France)

Rheumatology, vol. 7, pp. 11–18 (Karger, Basel 1982)

The Remodeling of Articular Cartilage[1]

Leon Sokoloff

Department of Pathology, State University of New York at Stony Brook, Stony Brook, N.Y., USA

Osteoarthritis is an inherently noninflammatory deformity of movable joints characterized by two discrete pathological processes: (1) deterioration and detachment of the bearing surface, and (2) proliferation of new osteoarticular tissue at the margins and beneath the detached joint surface. The sequences of these events are difficult to sort out because the process is ongoing and self-procreating. Three general concepts of these sequences have their own constituencies but seem to be overly simplistic (fig. 1).

(1) *Osteoarthritis is a degeneration of articular cartilage that progressively leads to denudation of the joint surface.* If this were valid, little or no remodeling of the bone should occur. Only rarely is this the case, and usually it is the consequence of antecedent inflammation or metabolic peculiarity in which mechanical abnormalities are absent.

(2) *Osteoarthritis begins as fibrillation of cartilage that leads to secondary remodeling of the bony components of the joint.* This is the common view. A principal difficulty is that one is hard put to isolate any individual finding as a unique morphological event that precedes others in the complicated changes seen in histological sections. It does not, for example, take into account the remodeling of the osteochondral junction as an early age-related change in cartilage.

(3) *Osteoarthritis is the consequence of changes in the stiffness of subchondral bone.* This view suffers the same limitations as the preceding.

It seem unrealistic to attempt to identify a unique initial event in the osteoarthritic process. What is important is that it is the structural disintegration of the osteoarticular junction and abrasion that lead to the loss of sub-

[1] Supported by grant AM 17258-06 from the National Institutes of Health.

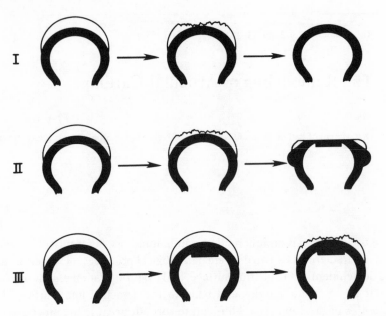

Fig. 1. Divergent concepts of the evolution of osteoarthritis. Bone is represented in black, and articular cartilage is the white cap upon it. Scheme I envisions the osteoarthritic process simply as progressive denudation of articular cartilage. In II, fibrillation of the cartilage is viewed as the first step. It leads ultimately to loss of bone at the articular surface as well as build-up of new bone beneath and at the margins of the joint surface. In III, the increase of subchondral bone precedes fibrillation of the cartilage.

stance of the articular surface (fig. 2). They also are responsible for the proliferative phenomena including the formation of new cartilage at the surface of the osteoarthritic joint.

Remodeling is the alteration of the internal and external architecture of the skeleton dictated by Wolff's law in response to variation in mechanical loading. It involves removal of bony tissue at certain points, while it is being laid down elsewhere. The concept has been expanded to the changes in the shape of joint with age and osteoarthritis. Analogous phenomena occur in soft connective tissues although they rarely have received systematic attention. Remodeling of articular cartilage must be regarded as one major aspect of the remodeling joint in osteoarthritis. Cartilaginous remodeling has three principal components: (1) structural removal of matrix; (2) formation of new cartilage, both its cells and matrix, and (3) endochondral calcification and ossification. These events are intimately associated with disturbances of mechanical forces acting on the joint surface. The purpose of this presenta-

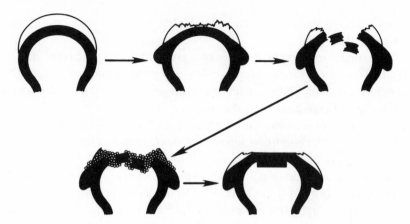

Fig. 2. Preferred view of osteoarthritic remodeling. Here fibrillation cannot be dissociated from remodeling of the mineralized tissue even in the earliest stages. The distinctive event is the disintegration of the osteoarticular surface, represented as depressed microfractures. It is in the reactive proliferation of new cartilage (bubbly material) and bone that the productive components of the deformity come about.

tion is to review some of the noteworthy advances that have taken place in our knowledge of the cellular and biochemical processes in the remodeling of cartilage. How they ultimately relate to the mechanical abnormalities is still unknown, but neither the biomechanical nor the cellular events can be ignored in evaluating pharmacological interventions in the management of degenerative joint disease.

Chondrolytic Mechanisms

The proteoglycans and collagen of the matrix are subject to proteolytic degradation through the synovial fluid or products of the chondrocytes themselves. Synovial cells and leucocytes in inflammatory exudates elaborate neutral proteases and collagenases as well as acid hydrolases [1].

The function of the latter in chondrolysis is unclear because the pH of the cartilage does not approach the optima of these enzymes. Chronic inflammatory changes are common in surgically resected specimens of synovium in osteoarthritis, but they usually are focal. Although the infiltrates are mild and probably of secondary or reactive nature, it is conceivable that inflammatory enzymes contribute to the destruction of the matrix. If this were the case, the destruction of cartilage in osteoarthritis should be diffuse. But it isn't.

Degradation of the matrix, even when widely dispersed in the tissue, characteristically is focal.

It is therefore more likely that degradation of the matrix in osteoarthritis results from short-range enzymes released by the chondrocytes into their immediate environs. Elevated levels of collagenase [2] and neutral proteases [3] in the cartilage have been documented chemically. Lysosomal enzyme activities also are elevated. They raise the possibility of an ancillary intracellular pathway for chondrolysis in the remodelling of this tissue.

The nature of the mechanical signal for the chondrocytes to digest their own matrix is unknown. Non-enzymic chemical messengers, called catabolins by *Dingle* [4], are elaborated by autolyzed synovium or activated macrophages. Catabolins are proteins having a molecular weight of about 20,000 daltons. They stimulate production of chondrolytic enzymes by chondrocytes in vitro. Access for messenger molecules to the chondrocytes is governed by the molecular sieve and ion-exchange properties of the matrix. Small peptides, free of carrier proteins, are thus more likely to enter the matrix than are larger ones. Some peptides act as enzyme inhibitors. Cartilage matrix contains such inhibitors. Of particular interest is a cationic anticollagenase (molecular weight $< 13,000$) that prevents penetration of the cartilage matrix by endothelial cells [5].

Cartilaginous Repair

Two avenues of repair of articular cartilage are permissible biologically: (1) replication of articular chondrocytes, and (2) metaplasia of granulation tissue that proliferates in the subchondral bone marrow and at the margins of the joint surface.

The traditional teaching that articular chondrocytes are incapable of mitotic division has been disproven definitively by cell culture studies. Clusters of chondrocytes in fibrillated cartilage represent clones of newly proliferated cells. The spaces the cells occupy constitute prima facie evidence of an associated chondrolytic process. Indeed a degree of chondrolysis seems to be a necessary condition for growth of the cells.

Cartilage formed by the second mechanism is an integral component of the osteophyte and also the reactive islets beneath the abraded joint surface. The new cartilage has a variously fibrous and hyaline character. At times the cartilage formation is extensive. Following osteotomies, much or all of the osteoarthritic joint has often been reported to be resurfaced by fibrocartilage.

Osteoarthritis therefore should be regarded not so much an inability but an aberration of the repair reaction of osteoarticular tissue.

Proliferation of Chondrocytes

Most of what is known about the control of growth of chondrocytes is derived from in vitro investigation. In culture, division of this cell type is anchorage-dependent. Although a specific attachment protein for chondrocytes – chondronectin – has recently been discovered [6], fibronectin also promotes this aspect of the proliferative process. Both proteins are present in serum and serum is necessary both for growth and for chondrogenic expression of the cells. In addition, serum contains several powerful, chemically discrete pentides that stimulate DNA synthesis by chondrocytes [7]. These include epidermal growth factor (EGF) and platelet-derived growth factor (PDGF). Fibroblast growth factor (FGF) acts in a similar manner but is not known to be in serum. So too does a factor derived from cartilage itself (CDGF). It is not presently known whether CDGF is synthesized in or simply taken up and stored by the cartilage [8].

Of these, none is more potent than ascorbate over a limited range of concentrations. At levels of $0.2\,mM$, vitamin C has growth-promoting effect in cell culture and, in combination with chondrolytic proteases, in organ-cultured articular cartilage as well [9]. At higher concentrations, ascorbate is markedly cytotoxic. It is thus of interest that impairment of repair of articular cartilage has been reported in subscorbutic guinea pigs following injury to joints [10].

Proteoglycan Synthesis

Stimulation of cartilage matrix formation is by no means a concomitant of chondrocytic proliferation [11]. Insulin and the insulin-like growth factors (somatomedins) as well as PDGF do have large effects on increasing radiosulfate incorporation into macromolecules in serum-free cultures. These effects are effaced as the concentration of serum increases above 5% in the culture medium. Cartilage itself has an extractable factor, distinct from CDGF, said to favor glycosaminoglycan synthesis [12]. Under most other circumstances, there is an inverse relationship between DNA and proteoglycan synthesis. As cell proliferation is stimulated by levels of serum above 5%, by

EGF, FGF, CDGF [13], platelet lysate or bovine embryo extract, each incre-
ment of DNA in the culture results in a cell-for-cell reduction of radiosulfate
uptake. The obverse situation has been observed when chondrocytes are cul-
tured in the nonanchored state. The cells suspended in spinner bottles do not
divide but make large quantities of proteoglycans. The profile of the glycosaminoglycans and the molecular species of collagen formed in suspension
express the cartilaginous phenotype [14].

An exception is seen in the case of 0.2 mM ascorbate. Vitamin C
increases proteoglycan synthesis at the same time that it promotes growth.
This effect is not obliterated by large quantities of serum, as seen in the case
of insulin. Furthermore, much of the proteoglycan is deposited about the
cells and a true chondroid matrix is formed. Thus ascorbate at this concentration offers the most effective stimulation of growth and matrix synthesis of
any of the factors tested.

Endochondral Ossification

Much is known and much unknown about the mineralization of cartilage and the induction of bone at a molecular level. Calcification and vascularization of cartilage are ordinarily closely associated phenomena but the relationship is not obligate for either of them. One wonders why articular cartilage does not become entirely calcified in the first place. The character of the
proteoglycans the chondrocytes have synthesized is known to affect the preci-
pitation of calcium salts in vitro [15]. A curious toxic effect of certain antibiot-
ics (oxalinic and pipemidic acids) may ultimately be a useful biochemical
probe of the control of this aspect of the mineralization process. In juvenile
animals these compounds produce a lysis of cartilage matrix confined to the
region destined to delineate the epiphysis from the articular cartilage [16].

Of particular interest at this time is the recognition of a cationic protease
inhibitor in the cartilage that prevents the ingrowth of endothelial cells into
the matrix [5]. Angiogenesis-inhibiting factors are also found in other brady-
trophic tissues and one can only speculate whether the cartilage-derived factor is a product of the chondrocytes proper. The implications for disturbances
of growth in chondrodystrophies and in the control of endochondral ossification are great.

The osteogenesis-inducing action of collagen has been affirmed many
times empirically and currently is being put to clinical trial. This factor has
not been purified. It is surmised to be collagenous, but the exact configuration

and molecular character of the collagen involved are not known. Prostaglandins also have profound influences on both the productive and the resorptive aspects of bone metabolism.

Concluding Remarks

The step-by-step unraveling of the biochemical events in the remodeling of cartilage is already a remarkable accomplishment. It does not denigrate either the achievement or the significance of the findings to recognize their limitations.

The in vitro behavior of articular chondrocytes in monolayer culture departs in many ways from that in suspension and more so in explant culture. There are differences even in monolayer culture related to the age and the species of animal studied. The serum with which the nutrient media is supplemented makes an enormous difference in the effect of individual nutrients, hormones and growth factors on growth and matrix production. None comes to grips with the basic biomechanical signals involved in the remodeling of the joint surface.

It is a truism that one extrapolates from experimental data in whole laboratory animals to clinical problems with great caution. The jump from data obtained about chondrocytes in a particular culture regimen to the behavior of joints in living animals is even greater. This caveat has not always been taken into account in the literature on proposed rational drug treatment of osteoarthritis. It should be.

References

1 Barrett, A.J.: Which proteinases degrade cartilage matrix? Semin. Arthrit. Rheumatism. *11:* suppl. 1, pp. 52–56 (1981).

2 Ehrlich, M.G.; Houle, P.A.; Vigliani, G.; Mankin, H.J.: Correlation between articular cartilage collagenase activity and osteoarthritis. Arthritis Rheum. *21:* 761–766 (1978).

3 Sapolsky, A.I.; Keiser, H.; Howell, D.S.; Woessner, J.F., Jr.: Metalloproteases of human articular cartilage that digest cartilage proteoglycan at neutral and acid pH. J. clin. Invest. *58:* 1030–1041 (1976).

4 Dingle, J.T.: Catabolin: a cartilage catabolic factor from synovium. Clin. Orthop. *156:* 219–232 (1981).

5 Kuettner, K.E.; Pault, B.U.: Resistance of cartilage to normal and neoplastic invasion; in Horton, Tarpley, Davis, Mechanisms of localized bone loss, pp. 251–258 (Information Retrieval, Arlington 1978).

6   Hewitt, A.T.; Kleinman, H.K.; Pennypacker, J.P.; Martin, G.R.: Identification of an adhesion factor for chondrocytes. Proc. natn. Acad. Sci. USA 77: 385–388 (1980).

7   Prins, A.P.A.; Lipman, J.; Sokoloff, L.: Effect of purified growth factors on rabbit articular chondrocytes in monolayer culture. 1. DNA synthesis (submitted for publication).

8   Azizkhan, J.C.; Klagsbrun, M.: Chondrocytes contain a growth factor that is localized in the nucleus and is associated with chromatin. Proc. natn. Acad. Sci. USA 77: 2762–2766 (1980).

9   Krystal, G.; Morris, G.M.; Sokoloff, L.: Stimulation of DNA synthesis by ascorbate in cultures of articular chondrocytes. Arthritis Rheum. (in press).

10 Schwartz, E.R.; Leveille, C.R.; Stevens, J.W.; Oh, W.H.: Proteoglycan structure and metabolism in normal and osteoarthritic cartilage of guinea pigs. Arthritis Rheum. (in press).

11 Prins, A.P.A.; Lipman, J.; McDevitt, C.H.; Sokoloff, L.: Effect of purified growth factors in rabbit articular chondrocytes in monolayer culture. 2. Proteoglycan synthesis (submitted for publication).

12 Kato, Y.; Nomura, Y.; Daikuhara, Y.; Nasu, N.; Tsuji, M.; Asada, A.; Suzuki, F.: Cartilage-derived factor (CDF) 1. Stimulation of proteoglycan synthesis in rat and rabbit costal chondrocytes in culture. Expl Cell Res. 130: 73–82 (1980).

13 Klagsbrun, M.; Langer, R.; Levenson, R.; Smith, S.; Lilehei, C.: Stimulation of DNA synthesis and cell division in chondrocytes and 3T3 cells by a growth factor isolated from cartilage. Expl Cell Res. 105: 99–108 (1977).

14 Sokoloff, L.: In vitro culture of joints and articular tissues; in Sokoloff, The joints and synovial fluid, vol. 2, pp. 1–26 (Academic Press, New York 1980).

15 Pita, J.C.; Howell, D.S.: Microbiochemical studies of cartilage; in Sokoloff, The joints and synovial fluid, vol. 1, pp. 273–330 (Academic Press, New York 1978).

16 Gough, A.; Barsoum, N.J.; Mitchell, L.; McGuire, E.J.; De la Iglesia, F.A.: Juvenile canine drug-induced arthropathy: clinicopathological studies on articular lesions caused by oxolinic and pipemidic acids. Toxicol. appl. Pharmacol. 5: 177–187 (1979).

L. Sokoloff, MD, Department of Pathology, Health Sciences Center,
State University of New York at Stony Brook, Stony Brook, NY 11794 (USA)

Rheumatology, vol. 7, pp. 19–28 (Karger, Basel 1982)

The Epidemiology of Osteoarthritis

J.G. Peyron

Centre de rhumatologie, Hôpital Tenon, Paris, France

Osteoarthritis (OA) is clearly a multifaceted disease, as recalled by *Lequesne* in this symposium. It probably has subsets among which cases with inflammation could make up a fairly important group, as *Huskisson* et al. [1]. *Dieppe* [2] and *Peyron* [3] have recently insisted upon. Even the pathology of OA does not lend itself to a systematic description. It is likely that we are dealing with a heterogenous group of conditions, indeed interrelated and overlapping, but with widely varying etiological and pathophysiological mechanisms. As this group of conditions is, at the same time, very widespread and becomes extremely frequent in ageing populations, it allows and invites an epidemiological approach.

Epidemiological studies of OA were initiated after World War II in an endeavor to evaluate its social and economic consequences amid the general burden of rheumatic diseases. *Kellgren and Lawrence* [3a] in the early fifties performed the now classical studies on the British communities in Leigh and Wensleydale. The Atlas of Standard Radiographs [4] of arthritis, published in 1963, allowed the different observers to compare their readings, at least approximately. Most of these studies have been summed up by *Lawrence* [5] in his book, which appeared in 1977. Moreover, numerous surveys of selected groups of patients, or of individuals more specifically exposed to abuse of their joints, have been conducted on both sides of the Atlantic in a search for etiological factors.

A certain number of autopsy studies have also been made since the classical papers by *Heine* [6] in 1926 and *Bennett* et al. [7] in 1942. However, aside from the difficult question of grading the lesions, to which the method of *Meachim* of painting the cartilage with diluted indian ink has brought some help, the correlation of actual pathological changes with clinical signs is weak and the significance of cartilage lesions as to the existence of present or future OA is uncertain. Indeed the studies of *Byers* et al. [8], *Goodfellow and Bullough* [9] and *Meachim and Emery* [10] have demonstrated that many lesions, especially in joint surface areas which usually do not bear weight, though similar to those noted in overt OA, will remain clinically silent and cannot be equated with OA.

It must be mentioned that skeletal remnants can be examined for the presence of bony exposure on joint surfaces and peripheral osteophytes. Such enquiries have been made by *Jurmain* [11] and *Rogers* et al. [12] and bring some fascinating historical evidence about this very ancient disease.

General Prevalence of OA

All presently available data point out that OA is extremely widespread with a high rate of prevalence in all regions of the world and in all ethnic groups. Generally speaking 1 or 2 adults out of 3, above 35 years of age, will display some degree of OA in at least one joint. *Lawrence and Sebo* [13] have compared the prevalence of OA in 17 populations, black, Indian and white, urban and rural, living between the latitudes of Alaska and South Africa, and have shown that there was no significant difference between the figures for the different groups.

Discrepancies between the results are largely accounted for by the differences in the methods used in each survey, which range from X-rays of hands only to a comprehensive radiological study of many joints sometimes helped by clinical evaluation. Inter-observer variations should also be taken into account, so that the figures provided by different studies should be compared only with great caution.

Influence of Age

Statistical data largely confirm the trivial evidence that the prevalence of OA is linked with age. The results of the classical study by *Lawrence* et al. [14] in 1966 of the rural and urban populations of two British districts showed that definite OA occurred in 2% of women under 45, about 30% of those between 45 and 65, and 68% of those aged 65 and more. In men, the corresponding figures were 3, 24.5, and 58%, respectively.

The role of age in favoring the onset of OA could be explained by several mechanisms, practically all of which are still largely speculative. They comprise anatomical modifications of the joint contours, decrease in the mechanical properties of articular cartilage and, possibly underlying these alterations, changes in the biochemical components of the matrix or in the chondrocytes.

That the joints are incongruent and that this feature, at least in the hip where the mechanism is most demonstrative, is the result of a dynamic process actively maintained through a permanent pressure-dependent remodelling of the bone-cartilage junction has been well documented [15–18]. In elderly people, joint congruency is increased, which seems deleterious to the physiological dumping of weight-bearing stress by the articular cartilage.

Some features of the mechanical resistance of articular cartilage seem to alter with age. This applies to the tensile stiffness under high loads [19], a property which is abolished by pretreatment of the cartilage with collagenase. Moreover, *Weightman* et al. [20] have demonstrated an age-related fatigue failure proneness of older articular cartilage, which means that it will rupture after a smaller number of mechanical stresses than young cartilage.

These changes in the mechanical properties of ageing cartilages point to some alterations in the collagen network, likely at the level of intermolecular cross-links or of fibrillo-formation, or of collagen-matrix interaction, a field poorly understood at present.

At the biochemical level, remarkably few changes have been documented. *Venn* [21] reports a slight decrease in water content, about 5%, especially in the deep layers of the femoral head, while the total glycosaminoglycan content increases very slightly, mostly through an increase in keratan sulfate and chondroitin-6 sulfate which tends to predominate over chondroitin-4 sulfate [22]. It is of interest that all these changes are the opposite of those which are reported in early OA lesions.

The proteoglycan monomers of old articular cartilage tend to have a mean length slightly shorter than those of young cartilage, at the expense of the chondroitin sulfate-rich region, so that they are somewhat enriched in protein and keratan sulfate [23, 24]. At least one discrete proteoglycan subpopulation disappears in cartilage samples from 35–40 years upwards [25]. Its role is unknown. Finally the aggregation capacity of proteoglycan from older cartilage seems impaired [26] thus eventually compromising the mechanical resistance of the matrix.

However, taken as a whole, all these changes do not provide a framework that would explain a 'natural' susceptibility of older cartilage to OA. It is likely that in OA some major change occurs in the metabolic behavior of the chondrocytes, the mechanism of which is presently not understood.

Mechanical Factors in OA Inception

At least we do know that among the factors which seem to bring about this metabolic shift, mechanical abuse of the joint is often suspected either in the form of a traumatic insult or of chronic overuse. Indeed numerous epidemiologic studies have been looking into the possible relations of mechanical factors and the prevalence of OA. Many surveys point to an influence of chronic mechanical overuse on the frequency of OA in selected population groups.

In most studies an increased involvement of the right hand over the left one is apparent [27]. OA has been found to be more frequent in miners than in dockers [28], and in dockers than in civil servants [29]. Farmers have displayed an unusually high prevalence of OA of the hip of comparatively early onset in several studies [30, 31]. The same features also appeared in a population of retired athletes [32].

In a large group of outpatients submitted to a detailed questionnaire, those seeking advice in a rheumatology department had significantly more often indulged in protracted sports than those attending an internal medicine clinic [33]. In a population working in a weaving factory, the hand and finger joints which most frequently had OA involvement were those which were the more heavily taxed by the repetitive movement imposed by each type of job [34].

In a large skeletal survey comparing the remnants of several ancient and recent populations, *Jurmain* [11] found that the prevalence of OA in each group was related to the strength and heaviness of the physical strains the individuals in the group had to sustain.

However, other studies, mostly those of the Leeds group [35], bring some discordant evidence. Contrary to several previous studies, professional soccer players did not display an excess of OA of the knee, nor did a large group of female physical education teachers [35], except for those who had sustained a meniscal injury in which case the relation to OA was significant. Professional runners are not exposed to an excess of OA of the hip [36]. The ankle joint of athletes is spared from OA [37] except in the case of bony or ligamentous damage. In pneumatic drillers, formerly said to be exposed to OA of the elbow, close radiological scrutiny of 34 cases displayed only two mild cases of true OA [35].

Obesity could be thought of as favoring the onset of OA in the lower limbs and indeed such a relation has been disclosed between overweight and OA of the knee joint, especially in females [5]. There is no agreement at the hip level, some studies point to an excess of overweight patients in these cases [38], while another study could not find an excess of OA of the hip in severely obese patients [39]. It is possible that obesity reflects an associated metabolic disturbance, together with an increased plasma uric acid level as frequently occurs. It can also be associated with static abnormalities such as varus deformities of the knees.

Finally mechanical overuse of a normal joint, devoid of static, meniscal or ligamentous trouble, does not seem to carry a seriously increased chance of initiating OA. Contrarily, traumatic damage to the joint is clearly a factor of OA. However, the pattern of OA distribution seems to be somewhat influenced by joint usage.

Sex and Hormonal Status

The prevalence of OA is clearly related to sex. Slightly more frequent in males up to 45 years of age, it becomes consistently and clearly predominant in females from 55 years onwards. Moreover, female OA is characterized by increased multiple involvement and by a particular pattern of distribution.

Lawrence et al. [14] showed that, between 55 and 64 years of age, 47% of women and 29% of men displayed four OA joints or more. While interphalangeal locations, especially the distal ones, the first carpometacarpal joint and the knees make up the most typical constellation of OA in postmenopausal women, the involvement of the metacarpophalangeal joints, the hip, the wrist, is more frequent in men.

The fact that this female predominance occurs at about the time of menopause raises the question of the role of estrogens as a possible protective factor against OA. However, *Rogers and Lansbury* [40] found no difference in urinary excretion of gonadotrophic hormones between postmenopausal women with and without Heberden's nodes, and *Dequeker* et al. [41] were not able to prevent progress of OA in a group of women with OA of the fingers in whom long-term estrogen therapy was started 1 year after the menopause.

Evidence from spontaneous animal OA in predisposed mice strains is somewhat difficult to interprete. However, it is of interest that on an experimental post-meniscectomy model of OA in the rabbit, *Rosner* et al. [42] recently reported favorable results of a treatment with tamoxifen, an anti-estrogen.

Generalized OA

Among all the clinical types that can result from multiple joint involvement and its associated features, *Kellgren and Moore* [43] in 1952 singled out a particular clinical constellation made up of locations to at least three joints or groups of joints, among which the interphalangeal joints, along with a frequent past or recent history of transient benign episodes of inflammatory polyarthritis with increased sedimentation rate.

Subsequently several studies tend to confirm statistically the validity of this concept, which seems at present to be rather generally accepted, in spite of a few studies that show no clear segregation of cases with multiple involvement, and tend to consider them as the upper end of a random distribution [44].

The concept of generalized OA stands out all the more clearly if only cases with five locations or more are taken into account, suggesting influence of a systemic factor [13]. Interestingly, two different clinico-epidemiological types of generalized OA emerge, depending on its main location to the fingers [13].

The nodal type, so-called because its main feature consists in Heberden's nodes of the distal interphalangeal joints, predominates largely in women and displays a definite familial aggregation. The non-nodal type, where proximal interphalangeal involvement is the most striking clinical sign, is only slightly predominant in women and displays a lesser familial tendency, but is frequently associated with previous episodes of inflammatory polyarthritis, a somewhat accelerated sedimentation rate, an increased plasma uric acid and obesity. The general impression is that hereditory factors play a major role in the nodal type, whereas inflammatory factors are instrumental in the non-nodal type.

This difference is again noticeable in the main etiological factors statistically associated with both types of finger OA when they are studied singly. Heberden's nodes show a marked familial tendency, confirmed by twin studies, to the point that their heredity is compatible with *Stecher's* [45] hypothesis: transmission by a single gene, dominant in women and recessive in men.

In the proximal interphalangeal joints, inflammatory features are sometimes so prominent that a special clinical type has been described, usually referred to as erosive OA because of frequent small bony erosions of the epiphysis of the phalanges on the X-rays. In this type, inflammatory flare-ups eventually involving other joints may at times mimick polyarthritis, though the outcome is usually favorable with a disappearance of inflammatory episodes.

In cases of primary OA of the hip, some studies point to the likelihood of subsets significantly associated with particular etiological factors. *Cooke* [46], looking for immune complexe deposition in the joint tissues, found a group of cases having IgM and complement-containing complexes, an increased number of other joints involved, a mildly accelerated sedimentation rate, and a somewhat rapid progress.

It should be recalled that several of these features have been described by *Lequesne and Amouroux* [47] in the type of OA of the hip which they called 'rapidly destructive'. In another study *Marks* et al. [48] noticed that cases of OA of the hip with radiological concentric joint narrowing are very significantly more often associated with Heberden's nodes than cases with upper pole or medial narrowing. Taken as a whole, these studies suggest that there exist one or several subsets in OA of the hip where systemic factors, possibly altering cartilage resistance, are particularly prominent.

Finally this review of the causes statistically involved in the different types and locations of OA makes it very obvious that the weight of each one of these etiological factors is very different depending upon the joint involved and sometimes the clinico-radiological type of OA [49].

OA of the distal interphalangeal joints and the type of generalized OA associated with it – nodal generalized OA – is mainly governed by heredity, a female sex factor and age. Location to the proximal interphalangeal joints and the type of generalized OA associated with it is principally dependent on inflammation, past or present, as well as on age, the female sex and, to a certain extent, on obesity. OA of the first carpometacarpal joint is governed by sex and age.

On the contrary, all locations to the lower limbs, as well as those to the shoulder and the wrist, depend mostly on mechanical factors, either in the form of a gross anatomical defect or of minor joint derangement or of accidental injury to the point that age, however important, is not sufficient by itself to bring about OA in these locations.

In conclusion, that wide disparity in the etiological factors depending on the different types of OA again raises the question put at the beginning of this paper: what we presently call OA is probably a heterogenous group of joint degenerative conditions which we observe only the only in their latest stage, the final common pathway.

References

1   Huskisson, E.C.; Dieppe, P.A.; Tucker, A.K.; Cannel, L.B.: Another look at osteoarthritis. Ann. rheum. Dis. *38:* 423–428 (1979).
2   Dieppe, P.A.: Calcium phosphate crystal deposition and clinical subsets of osteoarthritis, in Peyron, Epidemiology of osteoarthritis, pp. 71–80, (Geigy, Paris 1979).
3   Peyron, J.G.: Inflammation in osteoarthritis. Review of its role in clinical picture disease progress, subsets and pathophysiology. Semin. Arthrit. Reumatism *11:* suppl. 1, pp. 115–116 (1981).
3a Kellgren, J.H.; Lawrence, J.S.: Osteoarthrosis and disk degeneration in an urban population. Ann. rheum. Dis. *17:* 388–397 (1958).
4   Atlas of Standard Radiographs: The epidemiology of chronic rheumatism, vol. 2 (Blackwell, Oxford 1963).
5   Lawrence, J.S.: Rheumatism in populations, (Heineman, London 1977).
6   Heine, J.: Über die Arthritis deformans. Virchows Arch. path. Anat. Physiol. *260:* 521–663 (1926).
7   Bennett, G.A.; Waine, H.; Bauer, W.: Changes in the knee joint at various ages. (Commonwealth Fund, New York 1942).
8   Byers, P.D.; Contepomi, C.A.; Farkas, T.A.: Postmortem study of the hip joint. Ann. rheum. Dis. *29:* 15–31 (1970).
9   Goodfellow, J.W.; Bullough, P.G.: The pattern of the ageing of the articular cartilage of the elbow joint. J. Bone Jt Surg. *49B:* 175 (1967).
10 Meachim, G.; Emery, I.H.: Cartilage fibrillation in shoulder and hip joints in Liverpool necropsies. J. Anat. *116:* 161–179 (1973).
11 Jurmain, R.D.: Stress and the etiology of osteoarthritis. Am. J. phys. Antrhop. *46:* 353–366 (1977).
12 Rogers, J.; Watt, I.; Dieppe, P.A.: Arthritis in Saxon and mediaeval skeletons (in preparation).
13 Lawrence, J.S.; Sebo, M.: The geography of osteoarthosis; in Nuki, The aetiopathogenesis of osteoarthritis, pp. 155–183 (Pitman, London 1980).
14 Lawrence, J.S.; Bremner, J.M.; Bier, F.: Osteoarthrosis. Prevalence in the population and relationship between symptoms and X-ray changes. Ann. rheum. Dis. *25:* 1–24 (1966).
15 Johnson, L.C.: Joint remodelling as a basis for osteoarthritis. J. Am. vet. med. Ass. *141:* 1237–1241 (1962).
16 Green, W.T.; Martin, G.N.; Eanes, E.D.; Sokoloff, L.: Microradiographic study of the calcified layer of articular cartilage. Archs Path. *90:* 151–158 (1970).
17 Lane, L.B.; Villacin, A.; Bullough, P.G.: The vascularity and remodelling of subchondral bone and calcified cartilage in adult human femoral and humeral heads. J. Bone Jt Surg. *59B:* 272–278 (1977).

18 Goodfellow, J.; Mutsou, A.: Joint surface incongruity and its maintenance. An experimental study. J. Bone Jt Surg. 59A: 446–451 (1977).

19 Kempson, G.E.: The mechanical properties of articular cartilage; in Sokoloff, The joints and synovial fluid, pp. 177–238 (Academic Press, New York 1980).

20 Weightman, B.O.; Freeman, M.A.R.; Swanson, S.A.V.: Fatigue of articular cartilage. Nature, Lond. 244: 303 (1973).

21 Venn, M.F.: Variation of chemical composition with age in human femoral head cartilage. Ann. rheum. Dis. 37: 168–174 (1978).

22 Hjertquist, S.O.; Lemperg, R.: Identification and concentration of the glycosaminoglycans of human articular cartilage in relation to age and osteoarthritis. Calcif. Tissue Res. 10: 223–237 (1972).

23 Inerot, S.; Heinegard, D.; Audell, L.; Olsson, E.E.: Articular cartilage proteoglycans in ageing and osteoarthritis, Biochem. J. 169: 143–156 (1978).

24 Bayliss, M.T.; Ali, S.Y.: Age related changes in the composition and structure of human articular cartilage proteoglycans. Biochem. J. 176: 683–693 (1978).

25 Peyron, J.G.; Stanescu, R.; Stanescu, V.; Maroteaux, P.: Distribution électrophorétique particulière des populations de protéoglycanes dans les zones de régénération du cartilage arthrosique et étude de leur collagène. Revue Rhum. Mal. ostéo-artic. 45: 569–575 (1978).

26 Perricone, E.; Palmoski, M.J.; Brandt, K.D.: Failure of proteoglycans to form aggregates in morphologically normal aged human articular cartilage. Arthritis Rheum. 20: 1372–1380 (1977).

27 Acheson, R.M.; Chan, Y.K.; Clemett, A.R.: Newhaven survey of joint diseases. XII. Distribution and symptoms of osteoarthrosis in the hands with reference to handeness. Ann. rheum. Dis. 29: 272–286 (1970).

28 Duthie, J.J.R.: Rheumatism in the working population; in Second Nuffield Conference on Rheumatism (Nuffield Foundation, London 1964).

29 Partridge, R.E.H.; Duthie, J.J.R.: Rheumatism in dockers and civil servants. A comparison of heavy manual and sedentary workers. Ann. rheum. Dis. 27: 559–568 (1968).

30 Louyot, P.; Savin, R.: La coxarthrose chez l'agriculteur. Revue Rhum. Mal. ostéo-artic. 33: 625–632 (1966).

31 Pommier, L.: Contribution à l'étude de la coxarthrose chez l'agriculteur. Profil clinique et étiologique. A propos de 245 dossiers de coxarthrose chirurgicale; thèse Tours (1977).

32 Desmarais, Y.: Hanche du sportif; thèse Paris (1971).

33 Boyer, T.; Delaire, M.; Beranek, L.; Lasserre, P.P.; Tekaia, M.; Kahn, M.F.: Un antécédent de pratique sportive est-il plus fréquent chez les sujets atteints d'arthrose? Une étude contrôlée; dans Peyron, Épidémiologie de l'arthrose, pp. 156–163 (Ciba-Geigy, Paris 1981).

34 Hadler, N.M.; Gillings, D.B.; Imbus, H.R.; Levitin, P.M.; Makuc, D.; Utsinger, P.D.; Yount, W.J.; Slusser, D.; Moskowitz, N.: Hand structure and function in an industrial setting. Influence of three patterns of stereotyped repetitive usage. Arthritis Rheum. 21: 210–220 (1978).

35 Wright, V.: Biomechanical factors in the development of osteoarthrosis, epidemiological studies; in Peyron, Epidemiology of osteoarthritis, pp. 140–146 (Ciba-Geigy, Paris 1981).

36 Puranen, J.; Alaketola, L.; Reltokalio, P.; Saarela, J.: Running and primary osteoarthritis of the hip. Br. med. J., pp. 424–425 (1975).

37 Funk, F.J., Jr.: Osteoarthritis of the foot and ankle; in American Academy of Orthopedic Surgery Symposium on osteoarthritis, pp. 287–301 (Mosby, St. Louis 1976).

38   Kraus, J.F.; d'Ambrosia, R.D.; Smith, E.G.; Van Meter, J.; Borhani, N.O.; Franti, C.E.;
      Lipscomb, P.R.: Epidemiological study of severe osteoarthritis. Orthopedics *1:* 37–42
      (1978).
39   Goldin, R.H.; McAdam, L.; Louie, J.S.; Gold, R.; Bluestone, R.: Clinical and radiological
      survey of the incidence of osteoarthrosis among obese patients. Ann. rheum. Dis. *37:* 349–
      353 (1976).
40   Rogers, F.B.; Lansbury, J.: Urinary gonadotrophin excretion in osteoarthritis. Am. J. med.
      Sci. *232:* 419–420 (1956).
41   Dequeker, J.; Burssens, A.; Creytens, G.; Bouillon, R.: Ageing of bone. Its relation to
      osteoporosis and osteoarthrosis in post-menopausal women. Estrogens in the post-meno-
      pause. Front. Hormone Res., vol. 3, pp. 116–130 (Karger, Basel 1975).
42   Rosner, I.A.; Malemud, C.J.; Goldberg, V.M.; Papay, R.S.; Moskowitz, R.W.: Therapeu-
      tic effects of estradiol and tamoxifen in experimental osteoarthritis. Trans. Orthop. Res.
      Soc. *6:* 268 (1981).
43   Kellgren, J.H.; Moore, R.: Generalized osteoarthritis and Heberden's nodes. Br. med. J.
      i: 181–187 (1952).
44   O'Brien, W.M.; Clemett, A.R.; Acheson, R.M.: Symptoms and patterns of OA of the hand
      in the Newhaven survey of joint diseases; in Bennett, Wood, Population studies of the
      rheumatic diseases, pp. 398–406 (Excerpta Medica, Amsterdam 1968).
45   Stecher, R.M.: Heberden's nodes. A clinical description. Ann. rheum. Dis. *14:* 1–10 (1955).
46   Cooke, T.D.: Immune deposits in osteoarthritic cartilage. Their relationship to synovitis
      and disease site and pattern. Semin. Arthrit. Rheumatism *11:* suppl. 1, pp. 111–112 (1981).
47   Lequesne, M.; Amouroux, J.: La coxarthrose destructrice rapide. Presse méd. *78:* 1435–
      1439 (1970).
48   Marks, J.S.; Stewart, I.M.; Hardinge, K.: Primary osteoarthrosis of the hip and Heberden's
      nodes. Ann. rheum. Dis. *38:* 107–111 (1979).
49   Peyron, J.G.: Epidemiologic and etiologic approach of osteoarthritis. Semin. Arthrit.
      Rheumatism *8:* 288–306 (1979).

J.G. Peyron, MD, Centre de rhumatologie, Hôpital Tenon, 4, rue de la Chine,
F-75970 Paris Cédex 19 (France)

Rheumatology, vol. 7, pp. 29–45 (Karger, Basel 1982)

Biochemical Changes in Cartilage Relevant to the Cause and Management of Osteoarthritis

D.S. Howell, J.C. Pita, J.F. Woessner, Jr.

University of Miami School of Medicine, Arthritis Division and US VA Hospital, Miami, Fla., USA

Introduction

This brief review will deal with topics of interest in the osteoarthritis research arena which, from a clinician's standpoint are obviously relevant to either current or future therapeutic measures. Biochemical research approaches now bridge a panorama of subdivisions in science and involve looking at cartilage with many new methods and techniques. These all have complexities and limitations critically reviewed elsewhere [1–13]. A subjective and editorialized viewpoint will be expressed here and seems appropriate on the present occasion. No attempt at completeness is possible and previous reviews are recommended [1–13]. In the following dissertation the ideas are grouped under two major currently popular concepts of the pathogenesis of most forms of osteoarthritis at least in respect to the end results in cartilage: (1) physically produced biomaterial failure and (2) cellular intervention in cartilage destruction.

The Biomaterial Failure Concept of Osteoarthritis

Some investigators take the viewpoint that cartilage is simply a biomaterial in a bearing responding to microtrauma and occasionally macrotrauma. The point at which osteoarthritis (defined here as aggressive deep cartilage erosions or fissures leading to the final syndrome of joint instability and joint functional failure) appears at a time which is dependent largely on the joint history. Among the factors which influence the actual time of joint failure are the biomaterial deviations in configuration and alignment due to its growth and development and a particular type of trauma in quantity and quality. Prevention of aggressive cartilage breakdown by this view would invoke measures to identify subjects at risk, and to study the effects on the joints of amounts or types of exercise of athletic or industrial nature, changing nutrition, growth plate injury or subchondral bone fractures, as discussed by *Radin* in this symposium, leading to the final irreversible stage of tissue injury. Multiple disturbances of growth plates and adult remodelling probably contribute to the onset of osteoarthritis, as for example, the pistol grip deformities, tibial bowing, acetabular bone thickening. Biochemical regulation of growth plate and adult remodelling certainly partially determine the nature of these deformities, but are too complicated and focal for current therapeutic approaches. Prospects are dim for applying biochemistry to this phase of the osteoarthritis problem. Since many persons who have bony abnormalities or bowlegs do not develop aggressive osteoarthritis lesions despite vigorous athletic careers, obviously, there must exist a wide variation in biomaterial durability in the general population. Future research will undoubtedly, at least in animal models, probe the newly discovered mechanical structures contributing to durability and seek out hereditary or developmental errors, which would have predictive value for a development of osteoarthritis.

There has recently been much interest of researchers in a possible etiological role for subsets of osteoarthritis by calcium mineral salts in articular cartilage, particularly by calcium pyrophosphate dihydrate in the middle zones of articular chondrocalcinosis and hydroxyapatite in the deep radial zone as a response secondary to remodelling of subchondral bone. These minerals are postulated to have a noxious action on chondrocytes following sufficient accumulation in cartilage; also hydroxyapatite crystal aggregates and calcium pyrophosphate crystals have been found in in vivo animal and in vitro cell culture studies to be phlogistic [work of *R. Schumacher, T. Huskisson, P. Dieppe and D. McCarty,* reviewed in ref. 6].

Although there is much more that must be learned about the complexities of cartilage biochemical structure, the actual knowledge of collagen (50% of its dry weight) and proteoglycans (10% of dry weight) have been remarkably elucidated over the last two decades, as reviewed elsewhere [12, 13].

The concept of the tight and loose collagen network has partly arisen from the careful studies carried out by *Maroudas and Holborow* [8]. The enormous proteoglycan molecules in articular cartilage are partly in the form of subunits and partly aggregates, all of which have been studied in detail in sev-

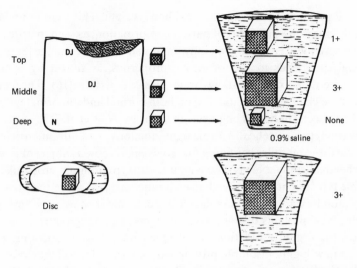

Fig. 1. Diagrammatic presentation of experiments [8] in which the hypothetical collagen network has been disrupted. The dissected pieces of osteoarthritic human cartilage from the middle zone were the earliest to swell when transferred to physiological solutions. The amount of swelling is exaggerated here for display purposes.

eral laboratories, such as those of *Muir, Hascall, Heinegård, Lowther, Sweet* and others. These molecules normally occupy large domains up to 50 ml/g dry weight when fully extended in solution. In hyaline cartilage they are constrained to far smaller volumes by the collagen network. There they form viscoelastic gels. Because of the high glycosaminoglycan content, they exert low hydraulic permeability. Thus, the amount of interstitial fluid lost from the surface of cartilage in the joint in vivo is limited under compression loads. When the load is removed, the layer of extruded lymph is reimbibed. The constraints on water imbibition imposed by the collagen network lead to at least 3 atm of pressure when the cartilage is unloaded. This figure increases proportionally to proteoglycan concentration during loading [8]. As pointed out by *Maroudas and Holborow* [8], the tight collagen network necessary to create this elastic mechanism in cartilage is demonstrable by the failure to swell and to imbibe water when pieces of fresh cartilage are placed in physiological saline (fig. 1). Also shown in figure 1 is the fact that, in contrast, normal nucleus pulposus does imbibe water, indicating a lack of a tight collagen network. It has been hypothesized that the difference compared to articular cartilage is due to the fact that proteoglycans are confined by the anulus fibrosus laterally and above, and below by the vertebral end-plates under considerable normal pressure of muscle tone and body weight. This rigid boundary framework causes the same sort of partial conformation, as seen in articular cartilage where there is a rigid wall only on one side of the cartilage [8]. Loss of proteoglycans leads to loss of elastic properties, as shown by several laboratories either experimentally or in diseased tissues [16]. The complexities of the changes in biomaterial on both normal and abnormal weight bearing have been studied in engineering terms by *Mow* et al. [17].

How collagen theoretically forms tight junctions at an ultramicroscopic level to constitute modules confining proteoglycans is now a subject of intensive biochemical study. Newly discovered hydroxypyridinium crosslinks of irreducible type might be involved at such junctions [18], since these crosslinks are found externalized in collagen bundles under some experimental conditions. New proteins distinct from collagen or proteoglycans might be candidates for a gluing function at collagen and collagen junctions. For example, a new highly insoluble protein with a molecular weight (MW) of 65,000 daltons has been discovered by *Paulsson and Heinegård* [19]. Chondronectin, a glue-like fibronectin may have some cement properties [20], and the calcium-binding protein of *Rosenberg* [21] needs similar studying in this role. Many other glycoproteins have been detected and need probing for a glue function at different cartilaginous sites.

The initial histological region in the cartilage of an osteoarthritic lesion is controversial. Possibly, there is deepening of cleavages from the cartilage surface cracks studied by *Gardner* [22], or, conversely, a deep separation of collagen bundles at their insertion into calcified cartilage has been documented and postulated to initiate disease [23]. Perhaps, there are varying initiation sites. The studies of *Maroudas'* group on histological layers tangentially sectioned from human osteoarthritic cartilage suggest that the collagen network often breaks earliest and the water content highest in the central region of osteoarthritic cartilage [8, 24]. This region would constitute the upper radial zone as well as the transient zone between vertically oriented and horizontally oriented collagen bundles of the tangential zone. Centrally located cystic lesions have sometimes been seen as an early osteoarthritic lesion. Inasmuch as the tangential zone is structurally braced to resist tensile forces and the radial zone compressive forces, it intuitively seems that at the interface of these zones, biomaterial vulnerability to various stresses might become manifest. Fiber network injury or cellular injury in this zone might account for the aforementioned findings of *Maroudas* as well as our findings in Pond-Nuki dog models of osteoarthritis, which by electron microscopy showed swelling of fibres and cell injury in central zones 4 weeks after initiation of the lesions [25]. More work is necessary to confirm or refute this viewpoint (fig. 1).

Recent studies by *Poole* et al. [26] support the hypothesis of a highly different biochemical architecture of a subtle nature exhibited by the tangential versus the radial zone interterritorial regions. Due to their very large size, hyaluronic acid-proteoglycan subunit link protein stabilized aggregates are anchored in the interterritorial region in the lattice work of the vertical collagen bundles [26]. Labelled antibody techniques have detected link protein almost entirely associated with the proteoglycans in this histological region [26]. In contrast, in the tangential zone and territorial matrix tissue around the cells, seemingly designed best for resisting tensile loads, the link protein was not associated with proteoglycan but irregularly spaced on collagen fibers. These findings either indicate the presence of unstable aggregates or the absence of aggregates of proteoglycans at such sites [26]. The actual 'free' space between collagen bundles seemed less in the territorial matrix where the collagen fibres are arranged in a more ordered parallel array and with more apparent proteoglycan association – a finding shown in several previous studies. It seems likely that some of the conformational properties conferred upon proteoglycans by hyaluronic acid in the aggregates might also be conferred upon them by the regular array of proteoglycans attached to the collagen surfaces or collagen-associated sugars or proteins. It also seems likely that among the determinants of proteoglycan aggregate size in a given cartilage site is the intercollagenous space to fill with conformed proteoglycan molecules. As shown by *Poole* et al. [26], the hyaluronic acid backbones span these spaces. Multiple intramolecular junctions with adjacent similar molecules are suggested to the observer by morphological data but have no biochemical backup as yet [27]. Some of the proteoglycans are resistant to extraction except by extreme methods, being bound in some manner within the collagen bundles, particular in the territorial matrix.

There is no time to describe a host of alternative hypothetical pathways involving biomaterial failure as the cause of osteoarthritis. A current popular viewpoint embodies fatigue failure of the collagen network or of those chemicals which glue or bond the collagen network together. Following such failure, proteoglycans no longer confined swell, imbibe water, unravel and extrude through erosions and fissures to the joint surface. Wear particles are carried to the lining membrane and a variable and low-grade inflammation develops. The presence of partially degraded or undegraded bits of cartilage containing type II collagen as well as mineral and proteoglycans has elegantly been demonstrated by a number of workers, most recently with a ferromagnetic technique by *Evans* et al. [28]. Among these constituents, mineral crystals are prominent. Evidence for an inflammatory role of hydroxyapatite clumps has been mentioned earlier [6]. The early loss of histological staining for sulfated proteoglycans could be due to changed proteoglycan conformation and swelling as well as lowered concentration through unravelling.

Because the collagen network and its constituents are so insoluble, it has been extremely difficult to test biochemically evidence of failure with aging. Indirect evidence of such biochemical failure is obtained, however, through biomaterial testing techniques with either indentation or tensile stresses placed on pieces of human cartilage studied as a function of aging. Significant reduction with aging was demonstrated in separate studies as well as softening and further losses in osteoarthritis lesions [29–31]. These reported changes with aging in normal cartilage, if correct for a general population, imply a premonitory weakening of the tissue prior to fatigue failure. This view was also supported in part by the findings, in two widely separated laboratories, in metabolic studies of incubated cartilage from osteoarthritic hips and knees. Namely, after incubation of precursors such as sodium ^{35}sulfate with the cartilage samples, there were no differences between osteoarthritis and normal controls in respect to rates of proteoglycan synthesis indices. Also, certain parameters of molecular size were not altered from normal in the osteoarthritic samples [32, 33]. Results of metabolic studies are somewhat at variance with work from some other laboratories, quoted below. Due probably to the sporadic temporal and histologic location of repair processes in osteoarthritis, to the difficulty of reproducible sampling, to the limitations of reporting, as discussed by *Maroudas,* and to the wide splay of data, this area of research has remained in a state of controversy [8].

The Cellular Intervention Concept

In this author's viewpoint, equally compelling evidence has accrued for a cellular role in the pathogenesis of most osteoarthritis seen with aging. The partisans of cellular intervention for the most part do not disregard as unimportant the developmental defects mentioned above or scoring of joints by physical trauma. Rather, the thesis is held that there is sufficient input into the process of cartilage breakdown by cellular products that therapeutic intervention in cell regulation might control the disease in many patients. This view offers much more chance for the medical therapy prior to the need for surgical intervention. This viewpoint is more of a hope than a fact, since, so far, administration of chemicals has not been shown to alter the course of osteoarthritis in humans. Limited alteration of progression with certain chemicals, however, has been shown in animal models. The biochemistry involved here does not emphasize faulty synthesis of the matrix or fatigue failure, but imbalance of normal cellular control mechanisms caused by a variety of etiological, usually extraneous mediators of physical or biochemical nature. The rapid disappearance of cartilage in human polychondritis in vivo [34] as well as the destruction overnight of proteoglycans and collagen within the cartilage matrix of samples treated in vitro with retinol or catabolin indicate the potential capability of chondrocytes to modify their matrix environment [35]. Although only 5–10% by volume of cartilage is comprised of chondrocytes [36], the potency of chondrocytic cathepsin B, D, F, neutral metalloproteoglycanase and serine neutral protease [35, 37, 38] as well as neutral collagenase [39–41] to destroy matrix components in a minute enzyme concentration in vitro is also devastating. The question arises, what mechanisms normally protect cartilage from harmful rapid breakdown? Which enzymes, if any, are participating in matrix slow turnover shown to be about 800 days in the human hip for a half-life of proteoglycans [8]? The collagen turnover normally is almost infinite, but speeds up under conditions of osteoarthritis at least in animal models. Which enzymes, if any, accelerate their function to destroy the cartilage matrix in osteoarthritis? Are oxygen-derived free radicals [42], as released in the course of lipid peroxidation, involved in proteoglycan or collagen breakdown? Among several laboratories which have a continuing interest in a possible cartilage enzyme action in the pathogenesis of osteoarthritis, there is a consensus based on documented studies that human cartilage is protected by potent endogenous inhibitors against some or all of the above neutral proteases [43–45]. Protection against the acid proteases of chondrocytes is provided by the lysosomal and plasma membranes. Only if the cells die, releasing these cathepsins from the lysosomes or other compartments, is there widespread chondrocytic coronal matrix damage, as seen in heated cartilage samples [10]. Thus, cartilage incubated with a potent inhibitor, pepstatin, or other inhibitors of cathepsin D, which permeate the matrix but not the living cells, blocks protease breakdown of dead but not living cartilage; and, therefore, it is assumed that cathepsin D is not instrumental in the breakdown of living cartilage, but rather other enzymes. Cathepsin D, acid phosphatase, cathepsin B, lysozyme and collagenase activities are frequently increased in the tissues of human osteoarthritis joints as recently reviewed [1–8]. Preliminary evidence for elevated neutral metalloprotease has been found. Unfortunately, the level of the free and total endogenous inhibitors for these enzymes has not yet been studied in cartilage. There are at least two further major uncertainties. First, the fact that cartilage matrix space must be hollowed out to accommodate cell multiplication in osteoarthritis provides an other reason for elevated proteases than to cause disease. This alternative explanation leaves involvement of extracellular matrix breakdown as an unnecessary accompaniment of the elevation of such degradative enzymes. Tissue remodelling would be well accomplished by extremely confined acid proteases such as cathepsin B, D, and F, which could function at the margin of the cells, and cathepsin D has been demonstrated and localized by immunological means to the edge of cell lacunae during cartilage breakdown in vitro [47]. Low pH necessary for these proteases to function could readily be developed at the edge of the cell hypothetically, but could not be attained $60 \mu m$ distant from the cell where the pH is probably 6.9–7.1. This leaves unexplained what enzyme makes the first breaks in the proteoglycans at distances from the cell beyond the reach of filopodia, which might extend less than $10 \mu m$. This reasoning led us to search for a neutral protease in chondrocytes. We have found over the last 10 years a neutral metalloprotease, which diffuses rapidly through cartilage and has some specificity for proteoglycan breakdown since it has no effect on casein or histone [37, 48]. Minute concentrations of this neutral protease in laboratory studies clip the proteoglycan subunits preferentially in the hyaluronic acid binding region (fig. 2), a finding similar to that of *Roughley and Barrett* [49] for some other proteases. Interestingly, on the other hand, in organ culture studies made during chondrolysis, some scientists have shown elaboration into the surrounding medium of proteoglycan subunits only slightly smaller than normal, as shown in figure 2. The proteoglycan subunits remaining in the whole tissue were of normal size and had not lost their capacity to combine to hyaluronic acid. Yet, almost all of those in the medium had lost this capacity [50, 51]. Degradation was blocked by neutral protease inhibitors and thereby diffusion of proteoglycans into the surrounding medium was prevented. How such large only slightly degraded molecules could diffuse through the matrix of the incubated cartilage pieces into the medium is an enigma. Globular proteins with an MW over 50,000 can hardly move into cartilage. One possible explanation of such movement is the presence of small channels arborizing in the matrix between the chondrocytes. A second view is based upon recent studies by *Cumming* et al. [52], indicating that elastic linear polymers can travel by facilitated diffusion through such a matrix, and fascinating evidence to support this view has been presented (fig. 3). It can be visualized without much imagination that in human

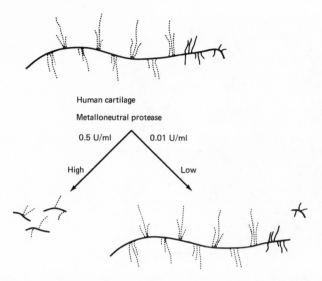

Fig. 2. Incubation for 5 h at 37 °C in synthetic lymph of human patellar cartilage neutral protease degraded proteoglycan subunits attached to hyaluronic acid (not shown) in aggregate form from about 25 to 19S in a diluted solution of enzyme, and from 25 to 3S in an undiluted protease preparation. Failure of reaggregation of this 19S product with hyaluronic acid indicated preferential breakdown of the hyaluronic acid binding region of the proteoglycan subunit. See text.

osteoarthritic cartilage a process similar to that observed in in vitro incubation could occur such that as fast mild proteolysis occurred these proteoglycans would diffuse into the synovial fluid and be even further degraded there or in the synovial lining. In this manner, at any one point in time almost no broken-down proteoglycans would ever be detected in the cartilage per se. Only the normal unbroken proteoglycans would remain selectively in the site, mostly attached to hyaluronic acid or collagen. Perhaps, subunits with an intact hyaluronic acid binding site are unable to diffuse as readily. These conjectures remain to be tested, it must be admitted. It has been suggested that, at least at certain times and at certain histological sites, accelerated proteoglycan turnover does occur in osteoarthritic cartilages in human as well as animal models [53–56]. What enzymes are involved in the degradation phase of this process remains to be determined. One explanation for the conflict of data is intermittency of the turn-on of such processes as well as certain differences in sampling and methodologies between laboratories. The recent findings of elevated active and latent collagenase in osteoarthritic human car-

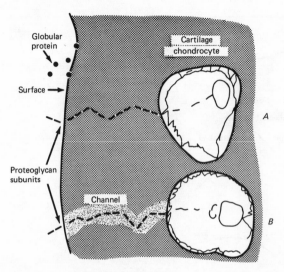

Fig. 3. Here is diagrammed the finding that slightly degraded proteoglycan subunits in organ culture appear to be elaborated into the synovial culture medium. Globular proteins when they weigh over 50,000 daltons diffuse extremely slowly into cartilage; elastic linear polymers may travel rapidly through gels by facilitated diffusion (A). Another view is that as yet undiscovered channels may exist in cartilage for passage of these still large slightly degraded proteoglycan molecules, > 1 million daltons (B).

tilage together with peptide fragments TCA and TCB in the tissue strongly suggest that collagen cleavage has occurred in these osteoarthritic samples [40, 57].

Mediators Influencing Chondrocytic Proteolysis and Repair

Whether the disease process or intracollagenous remodelling is affected by the above proteases is a difficult question. Unfortunately, no readily administered nontoxic inhibitor effective against any of the enzymes studied has so far become available. To block selectively the enzyme activity as well as tissue damage would obviously constitute strong evidence for a protease role in the pathogenesis of osteoarthritis. A search has been made at various centers for mediators from cells outside the cartilage, which might turn on their destructive enzyme capacities. For example, lymphocyte-activating factor (LAF), mononuclear cell factor (MCF) [58, 59], osteoclast-activating factor have all recently been reviewed. A similar or identical factor, studied in

Cambridge by *Dingle* [60], has been named catabolin by this investigator. Catabolin seems to differ little or not at all from mononuclear cell factor, but has been studied particularly on cartilage as a target tissue. Interestingly, this factor (or one very similar) seems to turn on a metalloneutral proteoglycanase as well as collagenase when incubated with bovine and other articular organ cultures [61, 62]. An interesting observation is that minced or injured synovium releases the MCF-like factor. It has a low molecular weight (20,000) allowing for rapid permeation of cartilage, and is not believed to be engulfed by α_2-macroglobulin. α_2-Macroglobulin is abundantly present, of course, in synovial fluid and under most circumstances protects cartilage from direct breakdown by synovial fluid or synovial lining membrane proteases [63]. This factor, or MCF, has already been found in rheumatoid synovial samples, but whether it is present in osteoarthritic tissues or fluids has not been documented. It is possible that intermittent or sporadic release of such a factor could turn on enzymes instrumental for osteoarthritis, but at present no data survey this point. Other mediators in synovial membrane include connective tissue activation peptide produced in tissue by migrating lymphocytes or polymorphonuclear leukocytes as well as platelets. This factor can stimulate cartilage proteoglycan turnover in vitro and is a likely candidate for some of the repair phenomenon observed in osteoarthritis [64].

Pharmacological Biochemical Considerations

Recent studies also suggest that suppressed production of the MCF-like factor, suppression of collagenase elaboration by target tissue cells and the increase of protease inhibitors are all simultaneously caused by small concentrations of hydrocortisone or dexamethasone included in incubates of relevant tissue, i.e., cartilage cells and rheumatoid pannus [65] (fig. 4). It currently seems more likely that control of protease release from chondrocytes among the various competing agents available on the drug store shelf will be more effective through suppression of mediator systems than through direct protease suppression per se.

In the final diagram (fig. 5) one can appreciate that the biochemistry of prostaglandins, that is the cyclooxygenase and possibly the lipoxygenase pathways not discussed here, may also be important in osteoarthritis, not simply because they suppress synovial pathways of inflammation but possibly because of their mediator effects on cartilage cells. *Chrisman* et al. [67] have shown an elevation in arachidonic acid levels in the cartilage after a blow

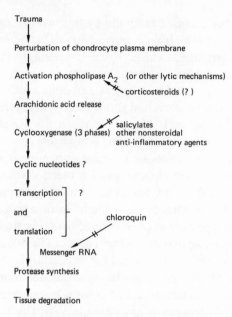

Fig. 4. Hypothetical cascade relating drug reaction to cartilage degradation [adapted from ref. 67, fig. 1].

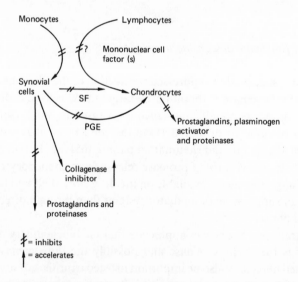

Fig. 5. Effect of corticosteroids based on tissue culture experiments, involving isolated articular chondrocytes, normal and rheumatoid synovial tissues in cultures [adapted from ref. 65, fig. 1].

Table I. Effect of mediators and a NSAID on $^{35}SO_4$ GAG synthesis in human osteoarthritic chondrocyte cultures [64]

	Stimulation, %
Additives	
0.15 *M* NaCl	–
CTAP[1]-I (lymphocytes)	37 ↑
CTAP-III (platelets)	104 ↑
CTAP-P_2 (platelets)	109 ↑
CTAP-I + Indocin (15 μg/ml)	16 ↑
CTAP-III + Indocin	51 ↑
CTAP-P_2 + Indocin	71 ↑

Although less so, the CTAP peptides are still effective on cartilage metabolism in the presence of Indocin, a neutral agent. Studies on negatively acting agents such as salicylates are needed.
[1] MWs 9–15 × 10^3 daltons and final concentrations 10–80 μg/ml.

on a dog patella simulating dashboard injuries. *Lippiello and Mankin* [66] showed that PGE and $PGF_{2\alpha}$ exogenously administered amplified the chondrocytic output of the same mediators in culture. Thus, aspirin and nonsteroidal anti-inflammatory agents as well as corticosteroids have been shown to influence favorably pathways which should hypothetically cause deleterious events in osteoarthritis. Currently, these nonsteroidal agents, for the most part, unfortunately also depress synthesis of proteoglycans in organ cultures of dogs and other cartilages [68]. Inhibition is less complete than with corticosteroids [69]. Further efforts to elucidate these in vitro findings and interpret them in in vivo situations are badly needed.

Perhaps, backup agents to block unfavorable cartilage responses from such agents would be a useful therapeutic approach in weight-bearing joints such as knees or hips. An example of what might be accomplished has been shown by *Castor* [64]. In his studies, the stimulatory effect of CTAP on proteoglycan synthesis and the partially sustained stimulation in the presence of a NSAID are shown in table I. A nontoxic stimulation of proteoglycan synthesis in vitro was also accomplished by ascorbic acid – an agent needing further study in this regard – in experimental osteoarthritis in guinea pigs [70]. Certainly, hopeful signs of improving the medical management of osteoarthritic patients over the next two decades may come from expanding biochemical research on the chondrocytic enzymes and mediators briefly reviewed here.

References

1   Brandt, K.D.: Pathogenesis of osteoarthritis; in Kelley, Harris, Ruddy, Sledge, Textbook of rheumatology, vol. 2, pp. 1457–1467 (Saunders, Philadelphia 1981).

2   Howell, D.S.: Biochemical studies of osteoarthritis; in McCarty, Arthritis and allied conditions; 9th ed., pp. 1154–1160 (Lea & Febiger, Philadelphia 1979).

3   Muir, H.: Proteoglycans: state of the art. Semin. Arthrit. Rheumatism *11:* suppl. 1, pp. 7–10 (1981).

4   Howell, D.S.; Moskowitz, R.W.: Introduction: symposium on osteoarthritis: a brief review of research and directions of future investigation. Arthritis Rheum. *20:* S96–S103 (1977).

5   Kempson, G.E.; Maroudas, A.; Weightman, B.: Conference on articular cartilage. Ann. rheum. Dis. *34:* suppl. 2 (1975).

6   Howell, D.S.; Talbott, J.H.: Osteoarthritis symposium. Semin. Arthrit. Rheumatism *11:* suppl. 1, pp. 1–147 (1981).

7   Peyron, J.G.: Epidemiology of osteoarthritis (Ciba-Geigy, Paris 1981).

8   Maroudas, A.; Holborow, E.J.: Studies in joint disease, vol. 1, 2 (Pitman, Tunbridge Wells 1980).

9   Nuki, G.: The aetiopathogenesis of osteoarthrosis (Pitman, Tunbridge Wells 1980).

10 Sokoloff, L.: The joints and synovial fluid, vol. 2 (Academic Press, New York 1980).

11 Howell, D.S.; Sapolsky, A.I.; Pita, J.C.; Woessner, J.F., Jr.: The pathogenesis of osteoarthritis. Semin. Arthrit. Rheumatism *5:* 365–383 (1976).

12 Howell, D.S.; Woessner, J.F., Jr.; Jimenez, S.; Seda, H.; Schumacher, H.R.: A view on the pathogenesis of osteoarthritis. Bull. rheum. Dis. *29:* 996–1001 (1979).

13 Gay, S.; Miller, F.J.: Collagen in the physiology and pathology of connective tissue (Fischer, New York 1978).

14 Kimura, J.; Thonar, E. Jo-M.; Hascall, V.C.; Reiner, L.A.; Poole, A.R.: Identification of core protein, precursor to cartilage proteoglycan. Semin. Arthrit. Rheumatism *11:* suppl. 1, pp. 11–12 (1981).

15 Pita, J.C.; Muller, F.J.; Howell, D.S.: Characterization of rabbit articular cartilage by rate-zonal centrifugation. Semin. Arthrit. Rheumatism *11:* suppl. 1, pp. 23–24 (1981).

16 Harris, E.D., Jr.; Parker, H.G.; Radin, E.L.; Krane, S.M.: Effects of proteolytic enzymes on structural and mechanical properties of cartilage. Arthritis Rheum. *15:* 497 (1972).

17 Mow, V.C.; Myers, E.R.; Roth, V.; Lalik, P.: Implications for collagen-proteoglycan interactions from cartilage stress relaxation behavior in isometric tension. Semin. Arthrit. Rheumatism *11:* 41–43 (1981).

18 Eyre, D.R.; Grynpas, M.D.; Shapiro, F.D.; Creasman, C.M.: Mature crosslink formation and molecular packing in articular cartilage collagen. Semin. Arthrit. Rheumatism *11:* 46–47 (1981).

19 Paulsson, M.; Heinegård, D.: Properties of a cartilage matrix protein. Semin. Arthrit. Rheumatism *11:* 14–15 (1981).

20 Martin, G.: Personal communication (1980).

21 Rosenberg, L.: Personal communication (1981).

22 Gardner, D.L.: Diseases of connective tissue: a consensus. J. clin. Path. *31:* S223–S238 (1978).

23 Meachim, G.; Bentley, G.: Horizontal splitting in patellar articular cartilage. Arthritis Rheum. *21:* 669–674 (1978).

24 Maroudas, A.; Venn, M.: Chemical composition and swelling of normal and osteoarthritis femoral head cartilage. Ann. rheum. Dis. *36:* 399–406 (1977).

25 Altman, R.D.; Tenenbaum, J.; Pardo, V.; Blanco, L.N.; Howell, D.S.: Morphological changes and swelling properties of osteoarthritic dog cartilage. Semin. Arthrit. Rheumatism *11:* 39–40 (1981).

26 Poole, A.R.; Pidoux, I.; Reiner, A.; Tang, L-H.; Choi, H.; Rosenberg, L.: Localization of proteoglycan monomer and link protein in the matrix of bovine articular cartilage: an immunohistochemical study. J. Histochem. Cytochem. *28:* 621–635 (1980).

27 Poole, A.R.: Unpublished observations (1981).

28 Evans, C.H.; Mears, D.C.; Cosgrove, J.L.: Secretion of neutral proteolytic enzymes by macrophages and synovial cells in response to wear particles in vitro. Trans. orthop. Res. Soc. *5:* 62 (1980).

29 Freeman, M.A.R.: Adult articular cartilage (Pitman, London 1978).

30 Kempson, G.E.: Mechanical properties of articular cartilage and their relationship to matrix degradation and age. Ann. rheum. Dis. *34:* S111–S113 (1975).

31 Weightman, B.: In vitro fatigue testing of articular cartilage. Ann. rheum. Dis. *34:* S108–S109 (1975).

32 Maroudas, A.: Metabolism of cartilaginous tissues: a quantitative approach; in Maroudas, Holborow, Studies in joint disease, vol. 1 (Pitman, Tunbridge Wells 1980).

33 McKenzie, L.S.; Horsburg, B.A.; Gosh, P.; Taylor, T.K.F.: Sulphated glycosaminoglycan synthesis in normal and osteoarthritic hip cartilage. Ann. rheum. Dis. *36:* 369–373 (1977).

34 Herman, J.H.: Polychondritis, chap. 91; in Kelley, Harris, Ruddy, Sledge, Textbook of rheumatology, vol. 2, pp. 1500–1508 (Saunders, Philadelphia 1981).

35 Barrett, A.J.; Saklatvala, J.: Proteinases in joint disease, chap. 14; in Kelley, Harris, Ruddy, Sledge, Textbook of rheumatology, vol. 1, pp. 195–209 (Saunders, Philadelphia 1981).

36 Stockwell, R.A.: Biology of cartilage cells (Cambridge University Press, Cambridge 1979).

37 Sapolsky, A.I.; Keiser, H.D.; Woessner, J.F., Jr.; Howell, D.S.: Metalloproteases of human articular cartilage that digest cartilage proteoglycan at neutral and acid pH. J. clin. Invest. *58:* 1030–1041 (1976).

38 Ehrlich, M.G.; Mankin, H.J.; Vigliani, G.; Wright, R.; Crispen, C.: Trans. 23rd Ann. Meet. Orthop. Res. Soc., 1977, p. 7.

39 Ehrlich, M.G.; Mankin, H.J.; Jones, H.; Wright, R.; Crispen, C.; Vigliani, G.: Collagenase and collagenase inhibitors in osteoarthritic and normal human cartilage. J. clin. Invest. *59:* 226 (1977).

40 Pelletier, J.P.; Martel-Pelletier, J.; Woessner, J.F., Jr.; Ghandur-Mnaymneh, L.; Enis, J.; Howell, D.S.: Direct measurement of cartilage collagenase activity in human osteoarthritis. Arthritis Rheum. *24:* S87 (1981).

41 Malemud, C.J.; Norby, D.P.; Sapolsky, A.I.; Matsuta, K.; Howell, D.S.; Moskowitz, R.W.: Neutral proteinases from articular chondrocytes in culture. 1. A latent collagenase that degrades human cartilage type II collagen. Biochim. biophys. Acta *657:* 517–529 (1981).

42 Greenwald, R.A.: The role of oxygen-derived free radicals (ODFR) in connective tissue degradation. III. Studies on hyaluronic acid (HA) depolymerization in inflamed synovial fluids (SF). Semin. Arthrit. Rheumatism *11:* 97 (1981).

43 Morales, T.: Unpublished observations (1981).

44 Keuttner, K.E.; Memoli, V.A.; Croxen, R.L.; Madsen, L.; Pauli, B.U.: Antiinvasion factor mediates avascularity of hyaline cartilage. Semin. Arthrit. Rheumatism *11:* 67–69 (1981).

45 Roughley, P.J.; Murphy, G.; Barrett, A.J.: Proteinase inhibitors of bovine nasal cartilage. Biochem. J. *169:* 721 (1978).

46 Sapolsky, A.I.; Malemud, C.J.; Norby, D.P.; Moskowitz, R.W.; Matsuta, K.; Howell, D.S.: Neutral proteinases from articular chondrocytes in culture. 2. Metal-dependent latent neutral proteoglycanase, and inhibitory activity. Biochim. biophys. Acta *658:* 138–147 (1981).

47 Poole, A.R.; Hembry, R.M.; Dingle, J.T.: Cathepsin D in cartilage: the immunohistochemical demonstration of extracellular enzyme in normal and pathological conditions. J. Cell Sci. *14:* 139 (1974).

48 Sapolsky, A.I.; Matsuta, K.; Howell, D.S.; Woessner, J.F., Jr.: Action of the neutral protease from human articular cartilage on proteoglycan. Arthritis Rheum. *22:* 655 (1979).

49 Roughley, P.J.; Barrett, A.J.: The degradation of cartilage proteoglycans by tissue proteinases: proteoglycan structure and its susceptibility to proteolysis. Biochem. J. *167:* 629 (1977).

50 Sandy, J.D.; Brown, H.L.G.; Lowther, D.A.: Degradation of proteoglycan in articular cartilage. Biochim. biophys. Acta *543:* 536 (1978).

51 Handley, C.J.; Lowther, D.A.: Extracellular matrix metabolism by chondrocytes. 5. The proteoglycan and glycosaminoglycan synthesized by chondrocytes in high density cultures. Biochim. biophys. Acta *582:* 234–245 (1979).

52 Cumming, G.J.; Handley, C.J.; Preston, B.N.: Permeability of composite chondrocyte-culture-millipore membranes to solutes of varying size and shape. Biochem. J. *181:* 257 (1979).

53 Mankin, H.J.; Dorfman, H.; Lippiello, L.; Zarins, A.: Biochemical and metabolic abnormalities in articular cartilage from osteoarthritis human hips. J. Bone Jt Surg. *53A:* 523–537 (1971).

54 Thompson, R.C.; Oegema, T.R.: Synthesis of proteoglycans in osteoarthritic human articular cartilage. J. Bone Jt Surg. *61A:* 407–417 (1979).

55 Mitrovic, D.; Gruson, M.; Demignon, J.; Mercier, P.H.; Aprile, F.; Deseze, S.: Metabolism of human femoral head cartilage in osteoarthrosis and subcapital fracture. Ann. rheum. Dis. *40:* 18–26 (1981).

56 McDevitt, C.A.; Muir, H.: Biochemical changes in the cartilage of the knee in experimental and natural osteoarthritis in the dog. J. Bone Jt Surg. *58B:* 94–101 (1976).

57 Axelsson, I.; Berman, I.; Howell, D.S.: Biochemical and electron microscopic characterization of rabbit articular and growth plate proteoglycans. Ass. Am. Physns, San Francisco 1981. Clin. Res. (in press).

58 Dayer, J.-M.; Krane, S.M.; Goldring, S.R.: Cellular and humoral factors modulate connective tissue destruction and repair in arthritic diseases. Semin. Arthrit. Rheumatism *11:* 77–80 (1981).

59 Dayer, J.-M.; Robinson, D.R.; Krane, S.M.: Prostaglandin production by rheumatoid synovial cells: stimulation by factor from human mononuclear cells. J. exp. Med. *145:* 1399 (1977).

60 Dingle, J.T.: The role of catabolin in arthritic damage. Semin. Arthrit. Rheumatism *11:* 82–83 (1981).

61 Ridge, S.; Oransky, A.L.; Kerwar, S.S.: Induction of the synthesis of latent collagenase and latent neutral protease in chondrocytes by a factor synthesized by activated macrophages. Arthritis Rheum. *23:* 448 (1980).

62 Phadke, K.D.; Lawrence, M.N.: Synthesis of collagenase and neutral protease by articular chondrocytes: stimulation by a macrophage-derived factor. Biochem. biophys. Res. Commun. *85:* 490 (1978).

63 Dingle, J.T.; Saklatvala, J.; Hembry, R.M.; Tyler, J.; Fell, H.B.; Jubb, R.W.: A cartilage catabolic factor from synovium. Biochem. J. *184:* 177 (1979).

64 Castor, C.W.: Synovial cell activation induced by a polypeptide mediator. Ann. N.Y. Acad. Sci. *356:* 304–317 (1975).

65 McGuire, M.K.B.; Meats, J.E.; Ebsworth, N.M.; Russell, R.G.G.; Murphy, G.; Reynolds, J.J.: Effects of corticosteroids on cellular interactions in human joint tissues in culture. Semin. Arthrit. Rheumatism *11:* 138–139 (1981).

66 Lippiello, L.; Mankin, H.J.: Positive feedback control of prostaglandin synthesis in articular cartilage. Trans. orthop. Res. Soc. *5:* 4 (1980).

67 Chrisman, O.D.; Ladenbauer-Bellis, I.M.; Fulkerson, J.P.: The osteoarthritic cascade and associated drug actions. Semin. Arthrit. Rheumatism *11:* 145 (1981).

68 Palmoski, M.J.; Colyer, R.A.; Brandt, K.D.: Marked suppression by salicylate of the augmented proteoglycan synthesis in osteoarthritic cartilage. Arthritis Rheum. *23:* 83–91 (1980).

69 Gray, R.G.; Tenenbaum, J.; Gottlieb, N.L.: Local corticosteroid injection treatment in rheumatic disorders. Semin. Arthrit. Rheumatism *10:* 231–254 (1981).

70 Schwartz, E.R.; Oh, W.; Leveille, C.R.: Osteoarthritis in guinea pigs: effects of vitamin C. Trans. orthop. Res. Soc. *5:* 214 (1980).

D.S. Howell, MD, Department of Medicine (D26), University of Miami,
School of Medicine, PO Box 016960, Miami, FL 33101 (USA)

Rheumatology, vol. 7, pp. 46–52 (Karger, Basel 1982)

Mechanical Factors in the Causation of Osteoarthritis

E.L. Radin

Department of Orthopedic Surgery, West Virginia University Medical Center, Morgantown, W.Va., USA

As far as the etiology of osteoarthrosis is concerned it would seem as the situation is getting more complicated and we know more and more about less and less. I suggest to you that what has happened over the past decade is instead of a group of experts, blindfolded, trying to describe an elephant, they now realize they are dealing with many different animals in the zoo. Not only is an attempt being made to describe, without seeing completely, elephants but also giraffes and hippopotamuses. I refer of course to the realization that osteoarthrosis should no longer be considered a disease but a collection of conditions whose common manifestation is deterioration of joints by wear and tear, i.e. primarily mechanical means. A clear description of these subsets of osteoarthrosis is important in order to exclude certain groups of patients from the diagnosis of osteoarthrosis and call them what they really are, in most cases some form of primarily inflammatory arthritis. Such a division will greatly help to end the present confusion. The second important concept to keep in mind, is that pathologists are having great difficulty explaining the pathophysiology of osteoarthrosis since the pathological changes in the joints are focal. For example within the same femoral head, removed at the time of total joint replacement, one finds areas of cartilage which appear histologically normal. In the same joint there are areas where the cartilage has totally disappeared, so whatever is happening does not happen systematically to the whole joint. It is almost as if we cannot see the forest for the trees and when we look at the trees we find many different species: oak, maple, spruce, palm. Clearly, the focal changes in the joint cannot be the result of a systemic change otherwise they would be geographically equal. We must stop looking for primary metabolic alterations in cartilage, and consider what it is in particular areas of the joint that causes the deterioration of cartilage we call ar-

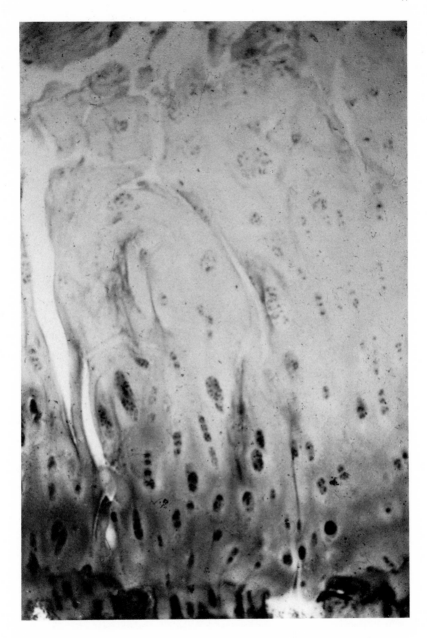

Fig. 1. Fibrillated cartilage. At the present time one cannot differentiate histologically between fibrillation which will be progressive or nonprogressive.

throsis. The third problem has been that the major focus of rheumatologic thinking is the role of inflammation. I think perhaps rheumatologists are at a disadvantage studying the pathophysiology of osteoarthrosis and arriving at a clear understanding, because their training focuses them on the inflammatory processes. I am pleased that everyone on this program believes that the inflammation in osteoarthrosis, although important, is secondary.

Figure 1 shows what is considered to be early fibrillation of articular cartilage. You probably still believe that fibrillation, once it begins in the joint is relentlessly progressive, finally going on to bare eburnated bone. That is not true. Fibrillated cartilage in certain areas of the joint survives very nicely. *Meachim* [1] was the first to point that out and the works of *Harrison* et al. [2], *Goodfellow and Bullough* [3] and our own work [4] have all shown that cartilage which is fibrillated, can survive for many years. We have now marvellous evidence from the Japanese [5, 6], using arthroscopic photography and cameras, showing us that in the same joint, over long periods of time, fibrillated areas which do not progress. The mere fibrillation of articular cartilage does not necessarily lead to osteoarthrosis. I define osteoarthrosis as osteoplyte formation and the loss of the cartilage substance, and I agree with *Leclerc's* definition. I think it is terribly important to keep that in mind. *Byers* et al. [7] pointed out that in the hip joint, articular cartilage in areas of the joint which are habitually unloaded tends to be nonprogressive and we know from the autopsy studies, which I already have eluded to [2–4], fibrillation in these areas is almost universal with age. Thus, we are dealing, in the joint, biochemically and histologically, with fibrillation, some of which is progressive and some nonprogressive, that it is difficult to tell apart. Progressive fibrillation tends to be in areas which are habitually loaded and to progress to bare bone and eburnation. Nonprogressive changes tend to occur in areas which are habitually unloaded and do not tend to progress. Thus, in order to start thinking clearly about the pathophysiology of osteoarthrosis, we must distinguish the softening and fibrillation of articular cartilage which does not necessarily progress.

I believe it is essential to discard from the subsets of osteoarthrosis, such as the Milwaukee shoulder, which are not in my view an arthrotic process but rather an arthritic or a primary inflammatory process. We did some studies on the patella, which almost universally shows areas of chondromalacia or nonprogressive fibrillation and also is subject to osteoarthrosis [4]. *Goodfellow* et al. [8] and *Meachim and Emery* [9] have also come to similar conclusions. What has been found in the patella is that the earliest fibrillation occurs on the central axes of the medial facet. It then can progress to a Collins grade

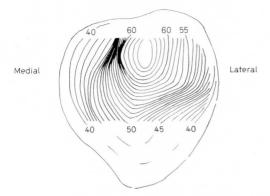

Fig. 2. Map of relative stiffness of patellar cancellous bone viewed from the articular surface. Note the steep stiffness gradient in the central-medial area. (Reprinted by permission. J. Bone Jt Surg. *60B:* 206, 1978.)

1 or grade 2 changes [10]. (Collins graded cartilage damage as I – superficial fibrillation; II – deep fibrillation; III – fibrillation to bone; IV – actual loss of cartilage substance with exposure of the subchondral bony plate.)

On the lateral patellar facet, when fibrillation occurs we initially cannot tell it apart, histologically from the medial side changes but the fibrillation on the lateral side will relentlessly progress. We have studied the bone, underneath these various areas of cartilage destruction. Figure 2 is a map showing the relative stiffnesses of the subchondral patellar bone. On the medial side one can see the sharp increase in relative stiffness of the underlying bone, this is a normal finding [4, 8]. It is precisely over this region that the universal chondromalacia (nonprogressive fibrillation) of the patellar articular cartilage initiates. Thus, one of the initiators of cartilage fibrillation is a steep stiffness gradient in the underlying subchondral bone, i.e., a place where the articular bed of bone abruptly changes in relative stiffness. In such an area one has relatively compliant bone juxtaposed to relatively stiff bone, creating a concentration of tensile stress. In such a structure the cartilage will tend to be ripped apart (fig. 3). Thus, fibrillation should be expected in such areas.

The absolute stiffness of the underlying subchondrial bone can play a great role in progressive loss of cartilage. We repeated *Meachim and Pedley's* [11] classic experiment of scarifying or making cuts with the scalpel in the surface of articular cartilage, in vitro, in joints which were oscillating and impulsively loaded, and, in some of these joints, we added a polymethylmethacrylate plug which stiffened the underlying bone about 20% [12]. We found, as *Meachin and Pedley* had, that simply scarifying the surface did not lead to

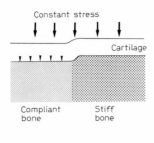

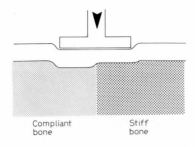

Fig. 3. Tearing (fibrillation) of cartilage will tend to initiate over areas of a steep stiffness gradient in the underlying bone, both under constant load or constant deformation. (Reprinted by permission. J. Bone Jt Surg. *60B:* 209, 1978.)

further loss of articular cartilage but that stiffening the bone did. I should emphasize that this is in the absence of enzymes. We are repeating this experiment in vivo and I hope to soon have the answer for you, enzymes and all. Our early results suggest the in vitro results occur in vivo as well. Cartilage wear off just over the area of the plug. One must conclude that the stiffening of the bone is a greater factor in promoting the loss of the articular surface than is fibrillation and in fact loss of cartilage can occur apparently without ever scarifying or purposely fibrillating the cartilage first.

I should like to report on another experiment [13], designed to see if 'overuse' created articular cartilage damage. We walked sheep on a concrete circular track daily for 2½ years, and at night, instead of putting them in a pasture we housed them on a paved parking lot. The control sheep were walked on woodchips and lived in grass pastures. We examined the knee joints of these two groups of sheep at the end of the 2½ years. The concrete-walked sheep clearly had an overusage of joints evident from the bony remodelling present, but they had no evidence of osteoarthrosis whatsoever. So it would appear that it is not how much you use the joint but the manner in which you use it that counts. We are currently embarked on a large study to look at the quantitative musculoskeletal shock absorption that occurs during the activities of daily living.

If you go back now and ask what are the factors that will lead to the progression of the cartilage change, we have found that cartilage fibrillation occurs in areas of the joint where the cartilage is subjected to a concentration of tensile stress. Not surprisingly cartilage will be torn (fibrillated) in areas where mechanical factors tend to tear it, particularly overlying steep gradients in subchondral bony stiffness, such as the edges of habitually contact and noncontact areas of most joints and in the case of the patella in the central medial facet region as well. Although this may not be the only cause of cartilage fibrillation it is certainly a proven cause. The progression of cartilage lesions to osteoarthrosis appears to require a relative stiffening of the underlying bone bed. We are currently investigating what can lead to this. Heavy work, in and of itself, does not make your joints wear out. Why do some of them wear out and others not is the critical question on which we are focusing our efforts.

Most importantly, it would appear as if the initiation and progression of cartilage lesions are two distinct phenomena. Studying the enzymatic, metabolic and histologic changes in articular cartilage in the process of deterioration, will not differentiate, at least at our present stage of sophistication, these two phenomena. Other factors are involved, probably mechanical, and the response of the living tissues to these different sorts of mechanical stress have not been well studied by traditional techniques.

Finally, it is important to remember that both inflammatory arthritis and mechanically induced arthrosis are common final pathways, not diseases. Remember, with our current level of understanding if you feel what seems like a hippopotamus it probably is a hippopotamus and you should not, for historical correctness, try to make an elephant out of it.

References

1 Meachim, G.: The effect of scarification on articular cartilage in the rabbit. J. Bone Jt Surg. *45B:* 150–161 (1963).
2 Harrison, M.H.M.; Schajowicz, F.; Trueta, J.: Osteoarthritis of the hip. A study of the nature and evolution of the disease. J. Bone Jt Surg. *35B:* 598 (1953).
3 Goodfellow, J.W.; Bullough, P.G.: The pattern of ageing of the articular cartilage of the elbow joint. J. Bone Jt Surg. *49B:* 175–181 (1967).
4 Abernethy, P.J.; Townsend, P.; Rose, R.M.; Radin, E.L.: Is chondromalacia patellae a separate entity. J. Bone Jt Surg. *60B:* 205–210 (1978).

5 Fujisawa, Y.; Masuhara, K.; Matsumoto, N.; Mii, N.; Fujihara, H.; Yamaguchi, T.Y.; Shiomi, S.: The effect of high tibial osteotomy on osteoarthritis of the knee. An arthroscopic study. Clin. Orthop. Surg. *11:* 576–590 (1976).

6 Fujisawa, Y.; Masuhara, K.; Shiomi, S.: The effect of high tibial osteotomy on osteoarthritis of the knee. An arthroscopic study of 54 knee joints. Orthop. Clin. North Am. *10:* 585–608 (1979).

7 Byers, P.D.; Contepomi, C.A.; Farkas, T.A.: A post mortem study of the hip joint. Ann. rheum. Dis. *29:* 15–31 (1970).

8 Goodfellow, J.; Hungerford, D.S.; Woods, C.: Patello-femoral joint mechanics and pathology. 1. Functional anatomy of the patello-femoral joint. J. Bone Jt Surg. *58B:* 287–290 (1976).

9 Meachim, G.; Emery, I.M.: Quantitative aspects of patello-femoral cartilage fibrillation in Liverpool necropsies. Ann. rheum. Dis. *33:* 39–47 (1974).

10 Collins, D.H.: The pathology of articular and spinal diseases (Williams & Wilkins, Baltimore 1950).

11 Meachim, G.; Pedley, R.B.: Topographical variation in patellar subarticular calcified tissue density. J. Anat. *128:* 737–745 (1979).

12 Radin, E.L.; Swann, D.A.; Paul, I.L.; McGrath, P.J.: Factors influencing articular cartilage wear in vitro. Arthritis Rheum. (in press, 1981).

13 Radin, E.L.; Orr, R.B.; Kelman, J.L.; Paul, I.L.; Rose, R.M.: Effects of prolonged walking on concrete on the knees of sheep. J. Biomech. (in press, 1981).

E.L. Radin, MD, Department of Orthopedic Surgery,
West Virginia University Medical Center, Morgantown, WV 26506 (USA)

Rheumatology, vol. 7, pp. 53–63 (Karger, Basel 1982)

Ultrastructural Approach to the Understanding of Osteoarthrosis

M. Carrabba[a], B. Colombo[a], E. Govoni[b], G. Cenacchi[b]

[a]IInd Chair of Rheumatology, University of Milan, Milan, Italy;
[b]Chair of Clinical Electron Microscopy, University of Bologna, Bologna, Italy

Ultrastructural studies on human articular cartilage in osteoarthrosis are scanty. Some investigations concerned the alterations of the surface [9], those of chondrocytes [12, 15], the aspect of the collagen fibres [4, 8] and the mineral content of the matrix [1, 2]. Other studies were devoted to general ultrastructural features [3, 5]. Most of these researches have outlined the presence of close morphological and functional links among the three main components of this tissue: chondrocytes, collagen fibrils (CF) and proteoglycans (PG). Thus, if a lesion is severe enough to irreversibly damage even one component, the others will alter and it is likely that the entire structure of cartilage will be soon disrupted.

In recent studies on the pathogenesis of osteoarthrosis a still unsolved problem concerns the component of the tissue which is first damaged by the different etiologic factors of this disease. The aim of this work was to elucidate some ultrastructural aspects of this problem comparing the main features of normal and osteoarthrotic human cartilage.

Materials and Methods

22 samples of femoral head cartilage were obtained from 22 patients with subcapital fracture (8 cases with normal cartilage) or with osteoarthrosis (14 cases) submitted to hip surgery (femoral head or total hip replacement). The mean age of the former group (controls, including 6 females and 2 males) was 69 years (range: 46–89), that of the latter (including 11 females and 3 males) was 64 years (range: 36–79). In each case, the sample (consisting of about half of the full thickness of the normal cartilage and removed from the most preserved areas of the osteoarthrotic femoral heads) was obtained in the course of the surgical treatment and immediately submitted to the following methods: (1) Fixation in glutaraldehyde, postfixation in OsO_4,

dehydration in ascending grades of ethanol and embedding in Epon to examine thin sections with transmission electron microscopy (TEM). (2) Fixation in glutaraldehyde, staining with Alcian blue plus $MgCl_2$ (0.9, 0.3 and 0.05 M) according to *Ruggeri* et al. [13], postfixation in OsO_4, dehydration and embedding in Epon to better examine PG with TEM. (3) Fixation in glutaraldehyde, dehydration in ascending grades of ethanol, drying with the critical point drying device and metallization with gold by the sputtering device to examine the samples with scanning electron microscopy (SEM). (4) Freeze with liquid nitrogen, fracture of the sample, replica of the fractured section by a carbon film according to the 'freeze-etching' method and examination of the obtained replicas with TEM.

Results

While in control samples the *surface* of articular cartilage examined with SEM presented a regular distribution of tertiary and quaternary hollows, that of osteoarthrotic samples was characterized by loss of such physiological depressions, unmasking of superficial CF, presence of empty lacunae and, in case of severe fibrillation, possible appearance of subchondral bone (fig. 1, 2). If the surface was examined by TEM, this zone appeared in control samples like a dense network of thin CF of similar diameter arranged tangentially to the surface (fig. 3); however, in samples from older subjects, the profile of this layer was often undulated (fig. 4). The study of the osteoarthrotic samples revealed the presence of numerous clefts deeply penetrating in the full thickness of cartilage and a diffuse infiltration of electron-dense material among CF of this zone (fig. 5). They appeared separated and partially hidden and began to exhibit an altered shape, size and capability of aggregation (more evident in the deeper zones) as demonstrated by the presence of some giant CF also in this layer.

The *chondrocytes* (which are flattened in the superficial zones and rounded in the intermediate) showed in osteoarthrotic samples two main alterations: (i) a degenerative reaction (prevailing in the superficial zones) including the various aspects of cell degeneration till necrosis and characterized by presence of cellular debris in the territorial matrix of the lacunae which were sometime filled with giant CF (fig. 6, 10), and (ii) a proliferative reaction with increase of number and sometimes with presence of fibroblast-like cells (fig. 7).

The *intermediate and deeper zones* showed with marked evidence the cellular alterations in osteoarthrosis, but those of the matrix were the most prominent. In particular, CF (which in these layers normally exhibit increased and more variable diameters than in the surface layers) presented

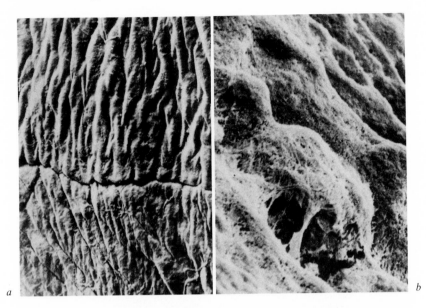

a   b

Fig. 1. Control articular cartilage (SEM). Secondary (*a*, ×1,500) and tertiary (*b*, ×3,400) surface undulations.

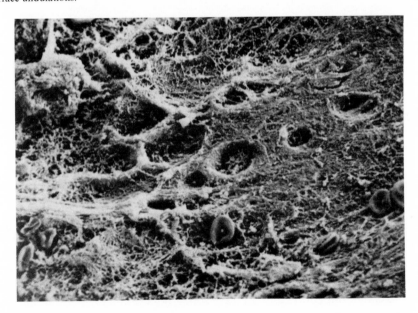

Fig. 2. Osteoarthrotic cartilage (SEM). Disappearance of physiological hollows, unmasking of CF and presence of surface erosions. ×7,000.

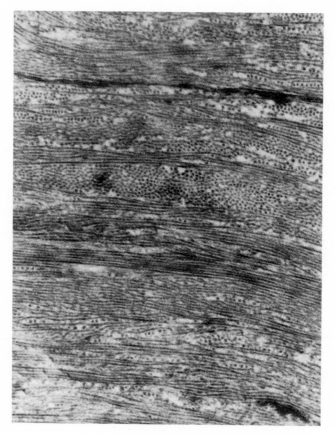

Fig. 3. Control articular cartilage (TEM). Little bundles of CF of the superficial zone. ×15,200.

a far more marked difference with thin fibrils often mixed with giant fibrils; the latter frequently showed signs of altered aggregation confirmed by the observation of flaked ends and by patterns of spirally arranged CF; finally, other CF exhibited an electron-dense material along their borders (fig. 8, 10). PG were clearly decreased in these samples, both in number and in size and such alteration, as shown with the Alcian blue method, seemed to involve mostly PG rich in chondroitin sulphate than those containing great amounts of keratan sulphate (fig. 9). In these zones, both cellular debris and the electron-dense material along the borders of some CF could represent a calcifying matrix (fig. 10).

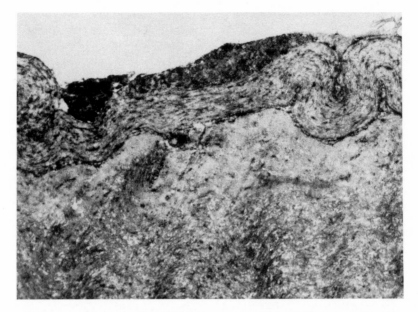

Fig. 4. Control articular cartilage (TEM). Presence of undulated CF on the surface of an old subject. × 4,900.

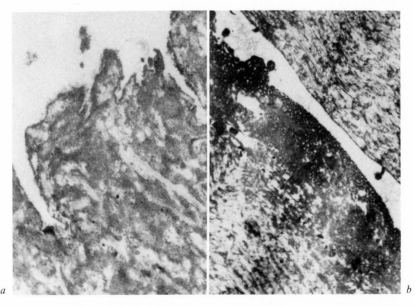

Fig. 5. Osteoarthrotic cartilage (TEM). Deep vertical cleft in fibrillating cartilage; the surface is infiltrated with electron-dense material. *a* × 15,000. *b* × 8,600.

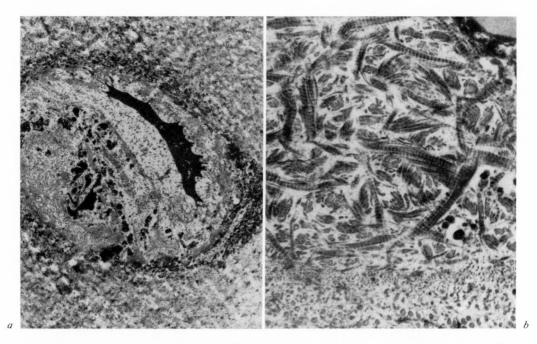

Fig. 6. Osteoarthrotic cartilage (TEM). Degenerated chondrocyte (*a,* × 5,000) and micro-scar (lacuna filled with giant CF; *b,* × 21,500).

Discussion

While some of our results add further details to the well-known osteoarthrotic lesions concerning chondrocytes and PG, others, although difficult to interpret, seem to enrich the actual data on this matter [14]. This is the case of the alterations of CF just described, which confirm previous studies [5, 8]. These lesions may be tentatively interpreted as a demonstration of reliability of the opinion of *Freeman* [7] and *Maroudas and Venn* [11] about a primary 'fatigue failure' of CF in osteoarthrosis. Other hypotheses, however, are possible: (i) a defect of chondrocytes of whatever origin (congenital, acquired or associated with an overload of their synthetic activity) with excessive release in the matrix of enzymes degrading both CF and PG [6], and (ii) an altered aggregation of CF depending upon an extracellular enzymic defect, an increased mineralization of the matrix [10] or an abnormal binding of PG with CF.

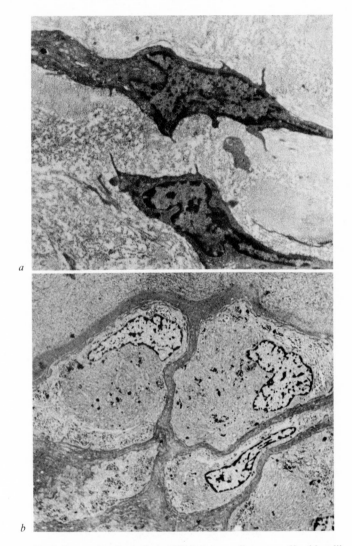

Fig. 7. Osteoarthrotic cartilage (TEM). Intermediate zone: fibroblast-like cells (*a,* × 7,200) and cluster of reactive chondrocytes (*b,* × 2,900).

The mechanisms of these processes and the role of articular cartilage and subchondral bone in their development are still obscure and have been largely discussed by the other investigators attending this symposium, but two points seem to emerge in recent years: the multifactorial origin of osteoarthrosis, and the central role of chondrocytes in this disease.

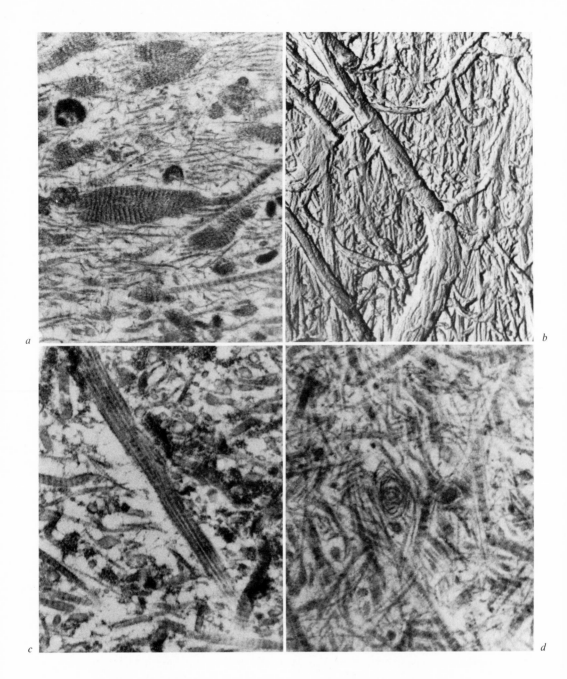

Fig. 8. Osteoarthrotic cartilage (TEM). Alterations of CF: marked difference in diameter (*a*, ×36,500); freeze-etching appearance of giant CF with flaked ends (*b*, ×18,700); altered aggregation of microfibrils running straight (*c*, ×25,000) or whirling (*d*, ×49,000).

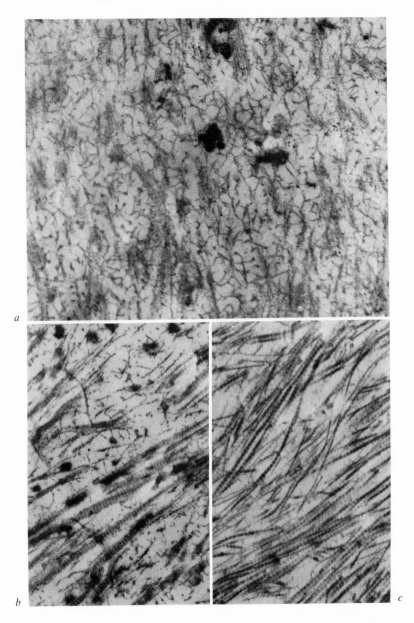

Fig. 9. Control articular cartilage (TEM). Aspect of PG in a sample treated with Alcian blue plus $MgCl_2$ 0.9 M (*a*, ×22,000). The beaded filaments (keratan sulphate-rich PG) are hardly decreased in osteoarthrotic cartilage (*b*, ×16,500), but are thinner if the sample is treated with hialuronidase beforehand (*c*, ×24,900).

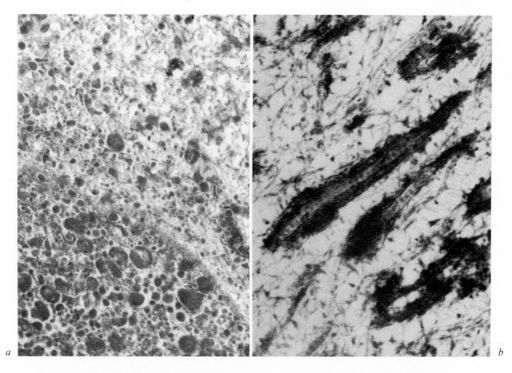

Fig. 10. Osteoarthrotic cartilage (TEM). *a* Cellular debris filling a lacuna and invading the territorial zone. ×12,300. *b* Sample treated with Alcian blue plus $MgCl_2$ 0.3 *M:* several CF are wrapped by an electron-dense alcianophil material. ×31,000.

We think that our results, although partial and provisional, are stimulating; further ultrastructural studies, however, are needed both in normal and osteoarthrotic cartilage to better clarify the importance of such approaches for the solution of the pathogenetic problems of osteoarthrosis.

References

1   Ali, S.Y.: New knowledge of osteoarthrosis; in Gardner, Diseases of connective tissue. J. clin. Path. *31:* suppl. 12, pp. 191–199 (1978).
2   Ali, S.Y.: Mineral containing matrix vesicles in human osteoarthrotic cartilage; in Nuki, The aetiopathogenesis of osteoarthrosis, pp. 105–116 (Pitman Medical, London 1980).
3   Ali, S.Y.; Wisby, A.: Ultrastructural aspects of normal and osteoarthrotic cartilage. Ann. rheum. Dis. *34:* suppl. 2, pp. 21–23 (1975).

4   Boni, M.; Monteleone, M.: Prime ricerche con il microscopio elettronico sulla cartilagine nell'artrosi deformante. Riv. Geront. Ger. *8:* 233–242 (1959).
5   Carrabba, M.; Colombo, B.; Angelini, M.; Cenacchi, G.; Govoni, E.; Marchini, M.: Aspetti ultrastrutturali della cartilagine articolare normale e artrosica. IV Congr. Latin de Rhumatologie, Liège 1980, Rapports, pp. 44–54 (Masson, Paris 1980).
6   Ehrlich, M.G.; Mankin, H.J.: Biochemical changes in osteoarthritis; in Nuki, The aetio-pathogenesis of osteoarthrosis, pp. 29–36 (Pitman Medical, London 1980).
7   Freeman, M.A.R.: The pathogenesis of idiopatic ('primary') osteoarthrosis. A hypothesis; in Nuki, The aetiopathogenesis of osteoarthrosis, pp. 90–92 (Pitman Medical, London 1980).
8   Ghadially, F.N.; Lalonde, J.-M.A.; Yong, N.K.: Ultrastructure of amianthoid fibers in osteoarthrotic cartilage. Virchows Arch. Abt. B Zellpath. *31:* 81–90 (1979).
9   Holt, P.J.L.: Joint cartilage. Physiology and changes in arthritis; in Holt, Current topics in connective tissue disease, pp. 24–47 (Churchill-Livingstone, Edinburgh 1975).
10   Howell, D.S.: Osteoarthritis. Speculations on some biochemical factors of possible aetio-logical nature including cartilage mineralisation; in Nuki, The aetiopathogenesis of osteoarthrosis, pp. 93–104 (Pitman Medical, London 1980).
11   Maroudas, A.; Venn, M.F.: Biochemical and physico-chemical studies on osteoarthrotic cartilage from the human femoral head; in Nuki, The aetiopathogenesis of osteoarthrosis, pp. 37–46 (Pitman Medical, London 1980).
12   Roy, S.; Meachim, G.: Chondrocyte ultrastructure in adult human articular cartilage. Ann. rheum. Dis. *27:* 544–558 (1968).
13   Ruggeri, A.; Dell'Orbo, C.; Quacci, D.: Electron microscopic visualization of proteogly-cans with Alcian blue. Histochem. J. *7:* 187–197 (1975).
14   Sokoloff, L.: Pathology and pathogenesis of osteoarthritis; in McCarty, Arthritis and allied conditions; 9th ed., pp. 1135–1153 (Lea & Febiger, Philadelphia 1979).
15   Stockwell, R.A.: Chondrocytes. Diseases of connective tissue. J. clin. Path. *31:* suppl. 12, pp. 7–13 (1978).

M. Carrabba, MD, Istituto Ortopedico G. Pini, IInd Chair of Rheumatology, University of Milan, Via Pini 3, I–20122 Milan (Italy)

Rheumatology, vol. 7, pp. 64–69 (Karger, Basel 1982)

Osteoarthritis: The Management
With 1 color plate

Israel Bonomo

Rheumatology Service, University Hospital, Faculty of Medicine, UFRJ, Rio de Janeiro, Brazil

In the management of osteoarthritis (OA), we all agree that we are fighting against the clinical picture of a disease which, until the present, has no cure. We want to emphasize the phrase, 'clinical picture', because it is well known and usual; the lack of relationship between radiological and clinical findings. Sometimes we register the worst radiological changes in asymptomatic joints.

Therefore, we should say that the clinical picture of OA is frequently, but not always, a result of a degenerative lesion of the joint cartilage. In this sense, it is important to remember some of the discrepancies observed in individual cases: (1) patients with closely related degrees of clinical pictures and X-ray changes; (2) severe clinical pictures with minimal (even absent), abnormal X-ray findings; (3) minimal clinical pictures with severe X-ray changes; (4) absence of complaints during prolonged periods (even years) in joints that have severe radiological changes that, in the past, were correlated with distressful disease, and (5) severe X-ray changes of joints, observed by chance, of individuals who always were and still are asymptomatic.

When looking at all these facts, we feel that, inspite of our ignorance regarding the causes and the measures to cure it, OA is not a hopeless disease. We should look for new ways which will lead to the state of clinical health.

Most of the new and old therapeutic measures for the treatment of OA are alphabetically listed below and looking at them we realize how confused those ways actually are: (1) acupuncture; (2) analgesics; (3) artificial lubricants; (4) aspirin; (5) cartilage and bone marrow extract; (6) exercise; (7) exogenous hialuronic acid; (8) heat; (9) hormones (tamoxifen); (10) intra-articular corticosteroids; (11) mucopolysaccharide polysulphuric acid ester; (12) NSAID; (13) orgatein; (14) reassurance; (15) surgery; (16) transcendental nerve stimulation; (17) weight reduction.

We still do not know why certain individuals have OA or why the joints of others with similar age, obesity and other physical and environmental factors remain clinically healthy. The prevention of this very frequent disease has been possible only in some forms of secondary OA. Good results may be obtained by the correction of genu valgum or genu varum, redirecting weight stress. The proper and early treatment of Legg-Perthes prevents some cases of secondary OA of the hips. It is also true that the correction of postural abnormalities of the spine will influence the appearence or severity of vertebral degenerative changes. But we do not know how to avoid secondary OA due to chondrocalcinosis, ochronosis or certain neurological disorders.

Recently the relationship between sports activities and degenerative joint diseases has been postulated by *Boyer* et al. Contradictory reports on jogging have appeared. Advanced degenerative changes of the knees, ankles and feet of football players are known by our colleagues specializing in sports medicine.

Since we are not succeeding in preventing OA, we should do our best in treating it. We endorse the feelings of many rheumatologists: OA, the result of a monotonous response of the cartilage to many factors, is not a single disease but a syndrome, and for its successful management we should look for ways of identifying its different forms.

Nowadays several treatments are planned in accordance with the different regional forms, such as Heberden's nodes, malum coxae senilis, gonarthrosis, etc., but for therapeutical purposes this simple classification in regional forms is not adequate. In the same regional form, for instance, we should identify secondary OA because the correction or elimination of its cause is fundamental.

Correction of axial misalignment (e.g. correction of genu valgum or genu varum by tibial or femoral osteotomy) may relieve pain giving a satisfactory result by stopping or retarding the progression of the disease. Other surgical procedures, like the removal of 'joint mice' and the debridement of a large osteophyte, could also help the patient. Hip arthroplasty (total hip replacement) and joint fusion are the surgical procedures widely accepted by orthopedists and rheumatologists for OA, with the problem that with fusion, motion is totally abolished. The merits of different techniques of knee arthroplasty are still being evaluated; therefore, until then all our efforts should be placed in medical treatment.

Even while looking for new procedures we should never forget that some patients only need very simple measures like reassurance and physical medicine (local heat and daily periods of exercise and rest), but the majority need drug therapy. It is also true that with the development of new drugs, the use and need of physical medicine has decreased.

The usual objectives of OA treatment are: (1) relief of pain (analgesics, rest); (2) regain motion (exercise); (3) correction of stressful deformities (surgery); (4) reduction of weight when weight-bearing joints are involved, and (5) avoidance of overuse (trauma). But the real objectives of treatment should be: (1) recognition of genetic predisposition; (2) elimination of the cause(s); (3) prevention of the primary lesion; (4) interference in the mechanisms of cartilage reaction and cartilage-synovium interactions, and (5) reversal of degenerative changes and stimulation of cartilage repair.

More emphasis should be given to the first four items, since there are many asymptomatic joints with advanced degenerative changes visible by X-rays.

We are not taking advantage of all the available clinical knowledge in evaluating drug effectiveness in OA of the knee. We have not seen one protocol, even in multicenter studies, that looks for the probable important subgroups, such as: (1) with or without valgum (or varus) deformity; (2) with or without significant difference in the length of lower limbs; (3) with or without obesity; (4) with or without degenerative changes of patello-femoral joint; (5) with or without degenerative changes of both tibial-femoral compartments; (6) with or without significant synovial effusion, and (7) with or without visible organic components of biological inferiority (flat feet, scoliosis, varicosity, spina bifida, sacralization).

As was said before, OA is not a disease but a syndrome and its diagnosis is made on a clinical basis. Therefore it is important to look for and to establish the subgroups.

The new therapeutic approaches look for symptomatic relief using drugs that act in the pathogenic mechanisms. Some drugs, such as cartilage and bone marrow extract which stimulate cartilage proteoglycan synthesis, are not widely accepted even after several years of use. Others, like artificial lubricants, are not very impressive.

It is our opinion that the major advance in the medical treatment of OA was the use of anti-inflammatory drugs that are responsible for the improvement to a variable degree of clinical symptomatology. Those who have used pure analgesics in the past have changed their prescriptions to a more effective symptomatic treatment – the anti-inflammatory agents. By this observa-

Table I. Total protein (g/100 ml) levels in synovial fluid of 15 cases of OA of the knees studied

Case	Total protein	Case	Total protein
21	2.2	30	3.7
15	2.5	27	4.0
19	3.1	28	4.1
23	3.3	9	5.0
24	3.4	10	5.6
25	3.4	26	6.6
13	3.5	22	6.6
20	3.6	Mean ± SD	3.89 ± 1.38

tion we are obliged to review and search for a role of a peculiar type of inflammation – 'dull', 'soft' – in the course of the disease. Much evidence suggests the existence of an inflammatory component that may be responsible for the clinical symptomatology. Not only pain, but local warmth can be detected by physical examination confirmed by thermography and diphosphonate scans. Morning stiffness and stiffness after sitting are usually reported and can be employed as a parameter of treatment effectiveness. Swollen joints are not unusual and synovianalyses disclose inflammatory findings which suggest the existence of more than one mechanism.

In the past we have examined the synovial fluid of OA knees and to our surprise found, in a group of 15 cases sequentially studied, that the total protein levels were higher than 3.0 g/100 ml. In the sample (table I) 3.9 g/100 ml was the arithmetic mean. Since then we have noticed several times the increase of total proteins (in one instance it was 11.3 g/100 ml).

Increased levels of immunoglobulins in the synovial fluid of OA patients have been reported. In a group of 12 cases we found an increase of 38% of IgG (665 mg%) 71% of IgA (103 mg%) and of 77% of IgM (71 mg%) (tables II, III). Only one of the 12 cases had normal levels of three immunoglobulin classes – IgG, IgA and IgM – (case 22) but we noticed, to our surprise, that this synovial fluid had large amounts of protein (6.9g%). In some cases, decreased levels of the complement were found due to the activation of the alternate or classical pathways. Rheumatoid factor detected by latex and Waaler Rose test were present in one third of the cases (5 of 15 cases) and antinuclear antibodies in only one.

So we think synovial analysis has shown much evidence of the presence of an inflammatory process. Arthroscopy also provides additional data and can clearly show inflammation of synovia and fibrilation of cartilage (fig. 1).

Table II. Synovial fluid levels (mg/100 ml) of immunoglobulins in 12 cases of OA of the knees

Case	IgG	IgA	IgM
19	940	148	50
20	600	124	100
21	780	64	100
22	460	64	24
23	640	112	80
24	448	100	66
25	100	176	60
26	400	64	140
27	600	112	44
28	840	102	44
29	440	74	44
30	840	100	100

Table III. Average amount of immunoglobulin in synovial fluid in OA

Ab class	Normal[1] (10 cases)	OA[1] (10 cases)	OA[2] (12 cases)
IgG	480	480	665
IgA	60	90	103
IgM	40	50	71

[1] Geiler, G.
[2] Bonomo, I.

Those who are engaged in the practice of rheumatology have observed the transitory but effective benefit of local injection of corticosteroids in the clinical symptomatology of OA. Even now, when many therapeutic measures are available, we, as many other physicians, utilize trials of intra-articular corticoid therapy in painful and stubborn OA joints. The results observed, sometimes dramatic, correlate well with the feeling of the existence of an inflammation.

New NSAID are yearly discovered in the continuous search for an ideal drug that will provide greater efficacy and/or better tolerance.

International acceptance of the use of anti-inflammatory drugs, instead of pure analgesic agents as a more effective symptomatic treatment of OA, has resulted in the inclusion of not only rheumatoid arthritis cases but also OA cases in the preliminary clinical trials of these new drugs.

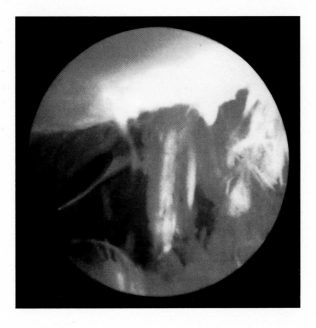

Fig. 1. Arthroscopy of an Osteoarthritic knee: inflammation of synovia and fibrillation of cartilage (courtesy of Dr. Katona).

We are far from reaching a satisfactory management of all the cases of OA and subsets have to be established. But with the use of anti-inflammatory drugs, the number of hopeless cases decreases and more patients become asymptomatic, even temporarily entering a state of clinical health.

Prof. I. Bonomo †, Head of Rheumatology Service, University Hospital, Faculty of Medicine – UFRJ, 21910 – Rio de Janeiro – RJ (Brazil)

Tiaprofenic Acid: Biology

Rheumatology, vol. 7, pp. 70–77 (Karger, Basel 1982)

Human Pharmacokinetics of Tiaprofenic Acid

J. Pottier, D. Cousty-Berlin, M. Busigny

Centre de Recherches Roussel–UCLAF, Romainville, France

Prior studies have shown that the oral absorption of tiaprofenic acid, partially gastric but mainly intestinal, is good in man, as in mouse, rat, rabbit, dog [1] and baboon [2]. It is markedly bound to plasma albumin and its apparent volume of distribution is small. Its plasma clearance is high, precluding any tissue retention. Of the two metabolic pathways, one leads to a phenol, from oxidation of the benzene ring in the para position to the ketone group, the other to an alcohol, from reduction of the ketone group. These metabolites are minor compounds in all species and are pharmacologically less active than the parent product [3]. Tiaprofenic acid is excreted partially conjugated as an amide in the dog and as an acylglucuronide in the other species including man. In animals orally dosed with ^{14}C-tiaprofenic acid, urinary excretion accounts for from one half of the ingested radioactivity in the rat to nearly 90% in the rabbit. In man, after hydrolysis of conjugates, the urinary excretion of tiaprofenic acid accounts for about 60% of an oral dose and that of its metabolites together for less than 5%.

In this paper, human plasma or serum kinetics of tiaprofenic acid are described after single oral, rectal, intramuscular or intravenous administration. In addition, steady state studies are carried out in the course of chronic oral or intramuscular treatment [4]. In some cases, urinary excretion of free and conjugated tiaprofenic acid was measured. Subjects of both sexes, without gastrointestinal, renal or hepatic diseases, were used. They were fasted overnight before oral or rectal administration. Tiaprofenic acid was administered as tablets, suppositories or as extemporaneous aqueous solutions of its tromethamine salt.

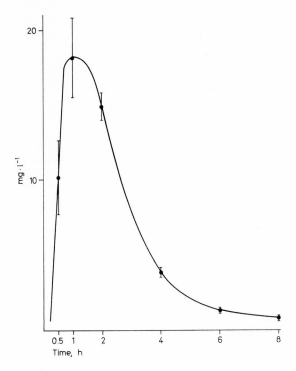

Fig. 1. Plasma kinetics of tiaprofenic acid after oral administration of 200 mg (mean ± SE, n = 9).

Plasma Kinetics and Urinary Excretion after Single Oral Administration

The subjects (n = 9, male, 24 years old, on average) received 200 mg of tiaprofenic acid. Mean plasma kinetics (fig. 1) shows that fast absorption occurs and high concentrations are reached 1 h after ingestion. Then the compound is rapidly cleared from the plasma. Pharmacokinetic parameters derived from compartment analysis are: lag-time (h), 0.32 ± 0.05; $t\frac{1}{2}$ abs. (h), 0.38 ± 0.05; C_{max} (mg·l^{-1}), 19.5 ± 2.5; T_{max} (h), 1.2 ± 0.1; $t\frac{1}{2}$ el. (h), 2.1 ± 0.3; Cl_p (l·h^{-1}·m$^{2-1}$) 2.2 ± 0.1. Urinary excretion of tiaprofenic acid (free and conjugated) for 24 h accounts for $57.3 \pm 5.3\%$ of the dose.

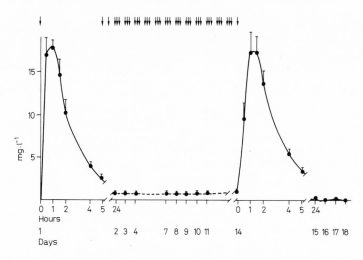

Fig. 2. Plasma concentrations of tiaprofenic acid during and after a chronic oral treatment with 600 mg/day (mean ± SE, n = 12). Arrows = Doses of 200 mg.

Plasma Concentrations during and after Chronic Oral Treatment

A daily dose of 600 mg, divided into three equal doses taken at 9.00 a.m., 2.00 p.m. and 8.00 p.m. was administered for 13 days to 9 male and 3 female subjects, average age 27 years. A 40th dose of 200 mg was administered on the morning of the 14th day. Plasma kinetics were determined after the first dose on day 1 and after the 40th and last dose on day 14. In addition, the residual levels were measured before the first daily dose on days 2, 3, 4, 7, 8, 9, 10, 11 and 14 and for 4 days after the end of treatment.

The kinetics after the first and the last administrations (fig. 2) exhibit similar profiles, the concentrations reaching 17 mg·l^{-1} on average and decreasing from 2 to 5 h according to identical apparent t$\frac{1}{2}$ of 1.5 h. The C$_{max}$ (20.7 vs. 20.0 mg·l^{-1}) and the areas under curves calculated from 0 to 5 h by the trapezoidal rule (44.4 vs. 49.0 mg·l^{-1}×h) do not differ significantly (paired t test). From day 2 to 14, the residual levels fluctuate from 0.6 to 1.0 mg·l^{-1} and, after the end of treatment on day 14, the concentrations are equal to or below 0.1 mg·l^{-1}.

This study confirms the rapid elimination and shows that the steady state is reached as early as the end of the first treatment day. Moreover the similar kinetics after the first and the 40th doses demonstrate that tiaprofenic acid cannot inhibit or induce its own biotransformation.

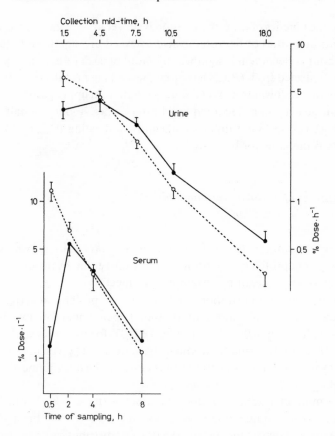

Fig. 3. Serum concentrations and urinary excretions of tiaprofenic acid after rectal (●, 300 mg) then oral (○, 200 mg) administrations to the same subjects (mean ± SE, n=9).

Serum and Urinary Excretion Kinetics after Single Rectal or Oral Administration

The same subjects (n = 9, female, 53 years old, on average) received 300 mg of tiaprofenic acid as suppositories then ingested 200 mg as tablets 2 days later. Serum concentrations, in percent of dose per liter, and urinary excretions, in percent of dose per hour, are shown in figure 3. There are not enough serum values to fit a curve and calculate pharmacokinetic parameters.

Serum concentrations 0.5 h after rectal administration are about one tenth of that recorded after ingestion, then they are slightly higher from 4 h.

In agreement, the kinetics of urinary excretion is slower after rectal than after oral treatment: quantities of tiaprofenic acid excreted are significantly less in the first 3-hour collection and significantly more in each of the three urinary fractions collected from 6 to 24h (paired t test). These results show that the absorption rate is slower from rectal mucosa than from upper gastrointestinal tract, but the excretions recorded in 24-hour urines, about one half of the dose in both cases, do not differ significantly, indicating that the total bioavailability is the same for both routes.

Serum Kinetics after Single Intramuscular or Intravenous Administration

Two groups of subjects (n = 5, female, both 45 years old, on average) received 400 mg of tiaprofenic acid (tromethamine salt) either by intravenous injection as reference route, or by intramuscular injection.

After intravenous administration, the kinetics of tiaprofenic acid (fig. 4) can be depicted according to a three-compartment open model with two distribution phases (t½ in h, 0.09 ± 0.01 and 0.54 ± 0.07, for the faster and the slower, respectively). Other pharmacokinetic parameters are given in table I. The apparent initial volume of distribution is close to plasma volume, 4.1% of body weight [5, p. 552].

After intramuscular administration, the kinetics (fig. 4, table I) can be depicted according to an initial diffusion or absorption phase from the injection site and a two-compartment open model (the fast distribution phase seen after intravenous injection is no longer apparent here). The diffusion is fast, without significant lag time and the peak appears 1 h after treatment. At this time, the concentration reached is close to that observed after intravenous injection. The elimination t½ and clearances are similar for both routes of administration.

Serum Concentrations during an Intramuscular Treatment for 2 Days

The subjects (n = 6, female, 46 years old, on average) received 1 intramuscular injection of 400 mg of tiaprofenic acid then 5 injections of 200 mg spaced out in 8-hour periods. Serum concentrations were determined 1 h after the 1st. 2nd, 4th and 5th administrations and just before each injection.

The concentrations (fig. 5) reached 1 h after the first injection (400 mg)

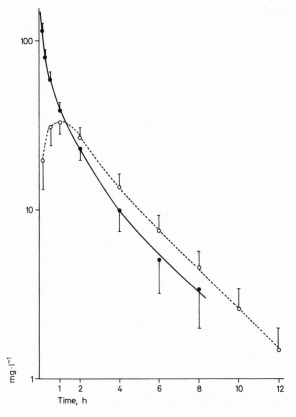

Fig. 4. Serum kinetics of tiaprofenic acid after intravenous (●) or intramuscular (○) injection of 400 mg (mean ± SE, n = 5).

Table I. Pharmacokinetic parameters of tiaprofenic acid (mean ± SE, n = 5)

	Intravenous	Intramuscular
C_o, mg·l^{-1}	155.4 ± 20.0	–
V_c, % of body weight	5.4 ± 0.4	–
t$\frac{1}{2}$ abs., h	–	0.28 ± 0.07
C_{MAX}, mg·l^{-1}	–	35.2 ± 5.5
T_{MAX}, h	–	0.98 ± 0.18
t$\frac{1}{2}$ el., h	2.29 ± 0.37	2.49 ± 0.24
Cl_p, l·h^{-1}·m$^{2-1}$ body area	1.82 ± 0.25	1.99 ± 0.25

t$\frac{1}{2}$ abs. = Absorption or diffusion t$\frac{1}{2}$; t$\frac{1}{2}$ el. = elimination t$\frac{1}{2}$; other symbols as in *Gibaldi and Perrier* [6].

V_c is expressed as percent of body weight and Cl_p as a function of body area calculated according to *Diem* [5, p. 642].

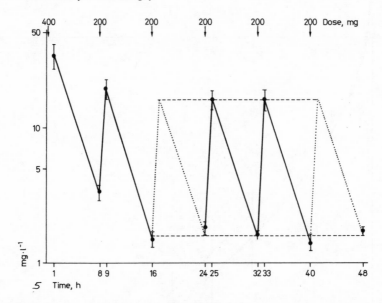

Fig. 5. Serum concentrations of tiaprofenic acid during intramuscular treatment for 2 days (mean ± SE, n=6). Arrows= Doses of 400 then 200 mg. – – –= Mean levels 1 or 8 h after injection of 200 mg; ········= simulated curves.

are similar to that recorded in a single administration of the same dose (33.9 vs. 36.4 mg·l⁻¹) and, 1 h after the 4th and 5th injections (200 mg), the concentrations are halved (16.0 and 16.1 mg·l⁻¹). The concentrations from 1 to 8 h after treatment (400 or 200 mg) decrease similarly with an apparent t½ of 2 h. From the 2nd injection, the residual levels measured 8 h after treatment fluctuate from 1.4 to 1.8 mg·l⁻¹. These results show that the steady state is reached as early as 16 h after the beginning of treatment according to this scheme.

To summarize, tiaprofenic acid is absorbed rapidly and efficiently from the gastrointestinal tract or from the intramuscular injection site, the plasma concentrations reaching 8–10% of the dose per liter 1 h after treatment. These high plasma levels indicate a small extravascular diffusion space, in agreement with initial apparent distribution volume close to plasma volume found after intravenous administration.

The absorption rate from rectal mucosa is slower than that from upper gastrointestinal tract, but the bioavailability is quantitatively similar for both routes. The elimination t½, about 2 h, and the plasma clearance, about 2 liters·h⁻¹ per m² of body area, rule out any risk of accumulation. Oral treatment for 2 weeks at a total dose of 8 g and intramuscular treatment for 2 days at a total dose of 1.4 g confirm this rapid elimination rate and show that the steady state is reached by the first day of both treatments. Moreover, chronic oral administration demonstrates that tiaprofenic acid does not inhibit or induce its own biotransformation.

References

1   Pottier, J.; Berlin, D.; Raynaud, J.P.: Pharmacokinetics of the anti-inflammatory tiaprofenic acid in humans, mice, rats, rabbits and dogs, J. pharm. Sci. *66:* 1030 (1977).
2   Chasseaud, L.F.; Down, W.H.: Metabolic fate of the anti-inflammatory drug tiaprofenic acid in the baboon. Report 5285-72-681 (Huntingdon Research Centre, Huntingdon 1972).
3   Clémence, F.; Le Martret, O.; Fournex, R.; Plassard, G.; Dagnaux, M.: Recherche de composés anti-inflammatoires et analgésiques dans la série du thiophène, Eur. J. med. Chem. Chim. ther. *9:* 390 (1974).
4   Pottier, J.; Cousty-Berlin, D.; Busigny, M.: Pharmacocinétique humaine de l'acide tiaprofénique. Reports AD54, AD95, AF11, AF58 and AG12 (Centre de Recherches, Roussel-Uclaf 1976–1978).
5   Diem, K.: Tables scientifiques; 6th ed. (Geigy, Basel 1963).
6   Gibaldi, M.; Perrier, D.: Pharmacokinetics; in Swarbrick, Drugs and the pharmaceutical sciences, vol. 1, p. 48 (Dekker, New York 1975).

J. Pottier, MD, Centre de Recherches Roussel-UCLAF, 111, Route de Noisy, F–93230 Romainville (France)

Rheumatology, vol. 7, pp. 78–87 (Karger, Basel 1982)

Pharmacological Profile of Tiaprofenic Acid

R. Deraedt, J. Benzoni, F. Delevallée

Centre de Recherches Roussel-Uclaf, Romainville, France

Many non-steroidal anti-inflammatory compounds have been used in the treatment of rheumatic diseases, but always with the same unsolved problem: the chronic administration of doses high enough to be really efficient without causing side-effects, especially in the gastrointestinal tract.

Tiaprofenic acid is 5-benzoyl-α-methyl-2-thiophene acetic acid (fig. 1), which appeared to be the most interesting compound in a series of alkyl derivatives of thienylacetic acids [1]. The pharmacokinetic study showed that its absorption was total in various species such as rat, mouse, rabbit, dog and human, that it was markedly bound to albumin and that its plasma clearance was high [2].

Mechanism of Action

The main characteristic of tiaprofenic acid is its remarkable inhibitory potency on cyclo-oxygenase, which transforms arachidonic acid into endoperoxides and then into prostaglandins (PGs). PGs are very important mediators of defence reactions and mainly of inflammation and pain, PGEs in particular potentiate the effects of other mediators such as bradykinin or histamine [3].

In vitro tiaprofenic acid was at least twice as active as indomethacin or diclofenac sodium and very much more so than ibuprofen in inhibiting PG synthesis from arachidonic acid by bovine seminal vesicle microsomes (fig. 2). When a guinea pig lung homogenate was used as the source of cyclo-oxygenase tiaprofenic acid was 10 times more active than indomethacin as an inhibitor.

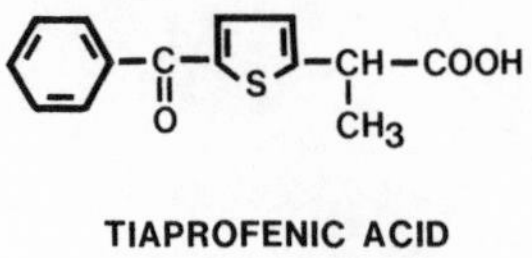

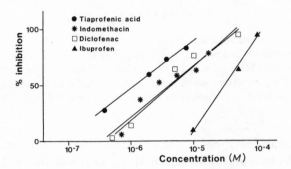

TIAPROFENIC ACID

Fig. 1. Tiaprofenic acid.

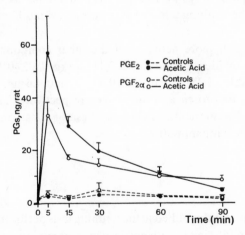

Fig. 2. Inhibition of PG synthesis in vitro. PG synthesis from arachidonic acid by bovine seminal vesicle microsomes for 30 min at 37 °C. PGE_2 and $PGF_{2\alpha}$ were measured by radioimmunoassay.

Fig. 3. Kinetics of PGE_2 and $PGF_{2\alpha}$ release in rat peritoneal fluid. Acetic acid was injected by i.p. route at the dose of 100 mg/kg in groups of 8–10 male rats weighing 200–250 g. PGs were measured by radioimmunoassay.

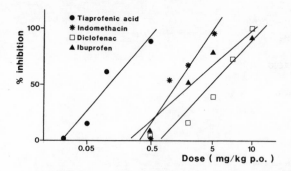

Fig. 4. Inhibition of PG release induced in the rat peritoneal fluid by acetic acid. Compounds were administered orally 30 min before acetic acid injection and PGs were measured 15 min after this injection. Mean PG levels were 1.5 ± 0.2 and 29.1 ± 3.6 ng PGE_2 per rat and 2 ± 0.2 and 16.6 ± 1.1 ng $PGF_{2\alpha}$ per rat for controls and acetic acid-injected animals, respectively, in 60 experiments. The inhibition was determined on the basis of the total PG level.

In vivo tiaprofenic acid also appeared to be at least 10 times more potent than indomethacin. We have previously shown [4] that acetic acid, the irritant used in the writhing test, injected into rat peritoneum provoked the release of considerable amounts of $PGF_{2\alpha}$ and even more PGE_2 into the peritoneal fluid with a peak as early as 5 min after injection (fig. 3). The inhibitory activities of the anti-inflammatory compounds on PG release were evaluated in this model of acute tissue pain: drugs were given orally 30 min before the injection of acetic acid, as in the writhing test, and PGs were measured 15 min afterwards.

Tiaprofenic acid was much more active than the other compounds (fig. 4): its ED_{50} (with 95% confidence limits) was 0.11 mg/kg (0.03–0.14) whereas it was 1.34 mg/kg (0.15–4.95), 2.2 mg/kg (0.3–7.3) and 4.6 mg/kg (2.0–12.4) for indomethacin, ibuprofen and diclofenac, respectively. This high inhibitory activity of tiaprofenic acid on PG biosynthesis or release may explain its strong action in acute inflammation.

Analgesic Activity

The analgesic activity was mainly studied in the writhing tests performed on mice or rats injected intraperitoneally with acetic acid or phenylquinone and treated with the drugs 30 min before this injection. In mice tiaprofenic acid exhibited a comparable activity in both tests: its ED_{50} values were

Table I. ED_{50} values (mg/kg p.o.) in the writhing tests

	Tiaprofenic acid	Indomethacin	Diclofenac	Ibuprofen
In mice				
Acetic acid	2.2 (0.3–4.8)	0.6 (0.5–0.8)	2.7 (1.4–6.3)	3.0 (1.2–5.3)
Phenylquinone	2.3 (0.2–4.6)	1.2 (0.7–2.2)	2.0 (1.0–3.0)	2.6 (2.4–2.9)
In rats				
Acetic acid	0.6 (0.1–6.6)	3.5 (1.4–12.2)		
Phenylquinone	0.3 (0.1–0.5)	5.8 (1.4–15.2)		

Writhing movements were counted during the 15 min following acetic acid (100 mg/kg) or phenylquinone (2.5 mg/kg) i.p. injection. Compounds were administered 30 min before the irritant. Groups of 10–30 female mice (weighing 20 g) or of 10–20 male rats (weighing 110 g) were used for each dose. In parentheses: 95% confidence limits.

2.2 mg/kg in the acetic acid test and 2.3 mg/kg in the phenylquinone test, doses very close to those of diclofenac and ibuprofen and slightly higher than that of indomethacin, with ED_{50} values of 0.6 and 1.2 mg/kg, respectively (table I). Tiaprofenic acid proved to be 3–4 times more efficient in rats than in mice, depending on the irritant used, whereas indomethacin on the contrary showed a weaker effect in rats (table I). This, as in PG release also measured in rats, the former compound was about 10 times more potent than the latter.

In the analgesic test in inflamed tissues, a modification of the method of Randall and Selitto, where the products were administered 4 h after the subplantar injection of yeast in rat hind paw, tiaprofenic acid increased the threshold of pain from the oral dose of 2 mg/kg. The ED_{100}, the dose which raises the pain threshold by 100%, was 20 mg/kg 30 and 60 min after treatment, while the ED_{100} for indomethacin was 5 mg/kg after 30 min and 10 mg/kg after 60 min.

On the other hand, in tests responding only to centrally acting analgesics, such as *hot plate* and *tail flick,* tiaprofenic acid displayed no effect at the high dose of 100 mg/kg orally like indomethacin at 50 mg/kg.

Anti-Inflammatory Activities

Anti-Oedema Activity. This was evaluated in various foot oedemas, differing by their intensity and their duration, provoked in the hind paw of rats by subplantar injection of different irritants or by a shock. The oedema

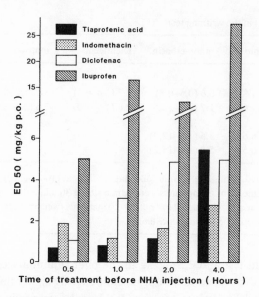

Fig. 5. ED$_{50}$ values in mg/kg p.o. in the NHA-induced foot oedema. Compounds were administered at different times before intraplantar injection of 1 mg NHA in a hind paw of male rats weighing 150–200 g. Paw volumes were measured before and 2 h after injection of the irritant. Groups of 8–16 rats per dose.

induced by naphtoylheparamine (NHA), which is short-lived and completely reversible in 24 h and concerns mainly the early phase of the inflammatory reaction, was measured 2 h after its production, while the oedema induced by carrageenin, which develops more slowly but is more long-lasting, was measured later, 5 h after the injection of the irritant.

Tiaprofenic acid was very active in the NHA-induced oedema: 3 times more so than indomethacin when administered 0.5 h before NHA: their respective ED$_{50}$ values were 0.57 and 1.77 mg/kg; it became less active than indomethacin only when administered 4 h before NHA (fig. 5). Indomethacin, therefore, appeared to have a more long-lasting effect. Diclofenac was less efficient, except when given 0.5 h before NHA, and ibuprofen even less so at all times of treatment.

In the carrageenin-induced oedema, however, tiaprofenic acid exhibited about the same action as indomethacin, their respective ED$_{50}$ values being 6.5 (3.3–18.3) and 4.9 mg/kg (3.6–8.1). Diclofenac was the most potent with an ED$_{50}$ of 2.3 mg/kg (1.5–3.7) whereas ibuprofen was the least active with an ED$_{50}$ of 36 mg/kg (19–60) (fig. 6).

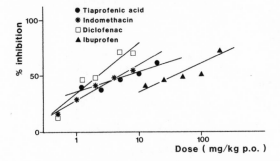

Fig. 6. Carrageenin-induced foot oedema. Compounds were administered orally simultaneously with the intraplantar injection of carrageenin (0.5 mg) in male rats weighing 150–200 g. Paw volumes were measured before and 5 h after injection of the irritant. Groups of 8–32 rats per dose.

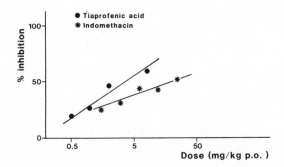

Fig. 7. Trauma-induced foot oedema. Trauma was provoked by the fall of a cylinder weighing 50 g from a height of 50 cm on the paw of male rats weighing 150–200 g. Compounds were administered orally immediately after this trauma. Paw volumes were measured before and 4 h after the trauma. Groups of 16 rats per dose.

On the other hand, in the traumatic oedema caused by dropping a weight onto the paw as described by *Riesterer and Jaques* [5], tiaprofenic acid showed the greatest potency (measurement 4 h after the trauma and the treatment): its oral ED_{50} of 3.6 mg/kg (1.8–32) was 5 times lower than that of indomethacin, which was 18.4 mg/kg (10.7–62) (fig. 7). Diclofenac exhibited only a slight effect at the high dose of 32 mg/kg and ibuprofen had no effect at the dose of 180 mg/kg. Thus in this oedema, where the vasomotor component may be very important as in the NHA-induced oedema, tiaprofenic acid also shows a high activity.

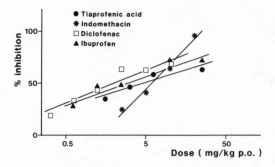

Fig. 8. UV erythema. Female guinea pigs were irradiated for 2 min on 3 spots 1 h after oral administrations of the compounds. The intensity of the erythema was evaluated 2 h after irradiation. Groups of 5–15 guinea pigs per dose.

Action in UV Erythema. In guinea pigs treated orally 1 h before being exposed to UV rays, the four compounds showed very similar activity 2 h after irradiation: the ED_{50} values were 4.7 (0.5–2.1), 5.8 (3.6–8.4), 2.0 (1.2–3.5) and 3.1 mg/kg (0.8–8.8) for tiaprofenic acid, indomethacin, diclofenac and ibuprofen, respectively (fig. 8).

Action in Adjuvant Arthritis. The drugs were incorporated in the feed of rats from the day of the intraplantar injection of the Freund-type adjuvant up to the 17th day (arthritis in development) or from the 15th to the 30th days (established arthritis). The intensity of the arthritis was expressed by an arthritic index based on primary inflammation, secondary inflammation and the serum level of α_2-macroglobulin.

In the arthritis in development, evaluated on the 17th day, tiaprofenic acid began to inhibit both primary and secondary inflammation at the dose of 1 mg/kg, indomethacin at 0.3 mg/kg, diclofenac at 0.5 mg/kg and ibuprofen at 23 mg/kg (fig. 9); ED_{50} values were then 4.6 (3.0–10.8), 0.8 (0.7–0.9), 1.2 and 66 mg/kg (34–143), respectively.

Higher doses were, of course, necessary to decrease the inflammatory events in the established arthritis; the ED_{50} values rose to 10.6 mg/kg for tiaprofenic acid, 1.2 mg/kg for indomethacin, and about 2 mg/kg for diclofenac and 100 mg/kg for ibuprofen.

Gastrointestinal Tolerance

The ulcerogenic effects of tiaprofenic acid were examined in acute tests both in starved rats for the action on the stomach and in fed rats for the action on the intestine. Indeed food and the entero-hepatic cycle play an important

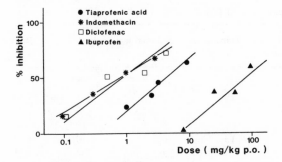

Fig. 9. Adjuvant arthritis in development. Groups of 10–20 male rats, 42–50 days old, were given an intraplantar injection of 0.10 ml of a Freund-type adjuvant (*Mycobacterium butyricum,* 6 mg/ml, in Bayol 55) and were sacrificed on day 17. The intensity of the arthritis was evaluated by an arthritic index taking into account primary inflammation, secondary inflammations and the serum level of α_2-macroglobulin. Compounds were incorporated in the feed from day 0 to day 17.

Table II. Ulcerogenic doses (mg/kg p.o.)

	Tiaprofenic acid	Indomethacin	Diclofenac	Ibuprofen
Gastric ulcer UD_{100}	47	9	10	170
Intestinal ulcer D_0	25	1	5	100
D_{100}	200	15	50	500

Gastric ulcers were evaluated in groups of 8–16 female rats weighing 130 g, starved for 24 h before treatment and sacrificed 7 h afterwards.
Intestinal ulcers were evaluated in groups of 8–16 male rats weighing 150 g, 24 h after treatment.

role in the appearance of intestinal lesions [6] and these lesions are observed in chronic toxicological experiments with non-steroidal anti-inflammatory agents.

For the *gastric lesions* recorded 7 h after oral treatment of rats starved for 24 h an index of ulceration was calculated, taking into account the mean degree of ulcer and the percentage of animals with ulcers; the UD_{100}, the dose corresponding to an index of 100, was determined: this was 47 mg/kg (25–218) for tiaprofenic acid, 9 mg/kg (4–19) for indomethacin, 10 mg/kg (7–13) for diclofenac and 170 mg/kg for ibuprofen (table II).

Intestinal lesions were evaluated 24 h after oral treatment. The maximum dose which did not cause any lesion in any of the rats (D_O) was 25 mg/kg for tiaprofenic acid whereas it was only 1 mg/kg for indomethacin,

Table III. Therapeutic indices: UD_{100}/ED_{50}

	Tiaprofenic acid	Indomethacin	Diclofenac	Ibuprofen
Acetic acid writhing	21	15	4	57
Phenylquinone writhing	20	7	5	65
PG release	427	7	2	77
NHA oedema (30 min)	82	5	10	35
Traumatic oedema	13	0.5	< 0.3	< 1
Carrageenin oedema	7	2	4	5
UV erythema	10	1.5	5	55
Adjuvant arthritis (in development)	10	11	8	2.5

Ratios of the UD_{100} or ulcerogenic dose in the stomach, and the ED_{50} values for the different analgesic and anti-inflammatory tests.

5 mg/kg for diclofenac and 100 mg/kg for ibuprofen. The minimum doses producing at least one ulcer in all animals (D_{100}) were 200, 15, 50 and about 500 mg/kg for tiaprofenic acid, indomethacin, diclofenac and ibuprofen, respectively (table II).

Thus the ratios of the ulcerogenic dose in the stomach and the different analgesic and anti/inflammatory ED_{50} values (UD_{100}/ED_{50}) give therapeutic indices which appear much better for tiaprofenic acid than either for indomethacin in all tests, except adjuvant arthritis, or for diclofenac in all tests. As regards ibuprofen, this has a higher index than tiaprofenic acid only for the writhing tests and UV erythema (table III). If we take the intestinal D_O for calculating this therapeutic index, all the indices are still more favourable for tiaprofenic acid by comparison with indomethacin and diclofenac.

Conclusion

Tiaprofenic acid proves to be a peripheral analgesic, which is slightly less active than indomethacin in mice but not in rats and equal in activity to diclofenac and ibuprofen. As an anti-inflammatory agent it is very active on acute inflammation; in oedemas such as NHA-induced oedema or traumatic oedema, it is the most potent of the four compounds studied. These results may be explained by its superior inhibitory action on PG synthesis or release. We have already observed [7] that inhibition of PG biosynthesis was mainly correlated with peripheral analgesic activity and activity on acute inflammation. It shows the same activity as indomethacin in other inflammatory models such as carrageenin-induced oedema and UV erythema, but is less active in adjuvant arthritis, a chronic model.

Since there is better gastric and intestinal tolerance to tiaprofenic acid than to indomethacin and diclofenac, the former has a higher therapeutic index. Thus, tiaprofenic acid should be of great value in the treatment of rheumatic diseases, since it is less limited than most of the non-steroidal anti-inflammatory compounds by its gastric irritant effects and should consequently be easier to handle. Moreover, by its remarkable activity on pain and acute inflammation it may be a very useful drug in osteoarthritis.

References

1   Clemence, F.; Le Martret, O.; Fournex, R.; Plassard, G.; Dagnaux, M.: Recherche de composés anti-inflammatoires et analgésiques dans la série du thiophène. Eur. J. med. Chem. *9:* 390–396 (1974).

2   Pottier, J.; Berlin, D.; Raynaud, J.P.: Pharmacokinetics of the anti-inflammatory Tiaprofenic acid in humans, mice, rats, rabbits and dogs. J. pharm. Sci. *66:* 1030–1036 (1977).

3   Ferreira, S.H.: Prostaglandins, aspirin-like drugs and the edema of inflammations. Nature, Lond. *246:* 217–219 (1973).

4   Deraedt, R.; Jouquey, S.; Delevallee, F.; Flahaut, M.: Release of prostaglandins E and F in an analgesic reaction and its inhibition. Eur. J. Pharmacol. *61:* 17–24 (1980).

5   Riesterer, L.; Jaques, R.: The influence of anti-inflammatory drugs on the development of an experimental traumatic paw oedema in the rat. Pharmacology *3:* 243–251 (1970).

6   Brodie, A.; Cook, P.; Bauer, B.; Dagle, G.: Indomethacin-induced intestinal lesions in the rat. Toxicol. appl. Pharmacol. *17:* 615–624 (1970).

7   Deraedt, R.; Jouquey, S.; Benzoni, J.; Peterfalvi, M.: Inhibition of prostaglandin biosynthesis by non-narcotic analgesic drugs. Archs. int. Pharmacodyn. Thér. *224:* 30–42 (1976).

R. Deraedt, Centre de Recherches Roussel-Uclaf, F-93230 Romainville (France)

Rheumatology, vol. 7, pp. 88–98 (Karger, Basel 1982)

Actions of Tiaprofenic Acid on Vascular Prostacyclin Biosynthesis and Thromboxane and 12-HPETE Formation of Human Platelets in vitro and ex vivo[1]

K. Schrör, V. Neuhaus, B. Ahland, S. Sauerland, A. Kuhn, H. Darius, K. Bussmann

Pharmakologisches Institut der Universität Köln, Köln, FRG

Introduction

Nonsteroidal anti-inflammatory drugs (NSAID) represent a group of chemicals that are used clinically for symptomatic treatment of inflammatory disorders. One property of these agents is their ability to inhibit the fatty acid cyclooxygenase and, thereby, the consecutive formation of prostaglandins (PGs) and thromboxanes (TXs) from free arachidonic acid (fig. 1). This observation, originally made by *Vane* [12] in 1971 initiated the synthesis of numerous compounds with the common feature of inhibition of cyclooxygenase and a proposed clinical use for treatment of symptoms, associated with inflammatory reactions [for review, see ref. 10].

Despite the apparent similarities in this basic mechanism, it is becoming more evident that there are differences between these agents which may be relevant also for the clinics. For example, NSAID may differ in their capacity to inhibit the cyclooxygenase of different tissues. Thus, it appears to be possible to inhibit the cyclooxygenase of blood platelets – a mainly TX and C-17 hydroxy acid (HHT) generating system – more easily than the enzyme in the vessel wall or sheep seminal vesicles, producing PGI_2 and PGE_2 as major cyclooxygenase-derived products [1, 8]. A dissociation between some NSAID was also found by comparing PGE_2 formation in inflammatory exudates with PGI_2 formation in stomach mucosa after oral administration to rats [13].

According to current knowledge, it would be useful to inhibit the biosynthesis of thromboxanes and HHT, a chemotactic compound for leuko-

[1] The measurements of the tiaprofenic acid serum levels were kindly performed by the Institut für Klinische Pharmakologie, Bobenheim (Prof. *Lücker*).

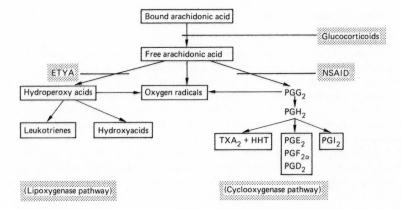

Fig. 1. Formation of products of arachidonic acid peroxidation during inflammation and its inhibition by drugs. *Glucocorticoids* prevent the release of arachidonic acid. Acetylene fatty acids *(ETYA)* inhibit the lipoxygenase pathway and formation of hydroperoxy and hydroxy acids, nonsteroidal antiinflammatory drugs *(NSAID)* inhibit the cyclooxygenase pathway and formation of prostaglandins (PGs), thromboxanes (TXs) and hydroxy acid (HHT).

cytes [4], while leaving PGI_2 formation unimpaired. PGI_2 and PGEs enhance the vascular symptoms of acute inflammation (vasodilation, exudation, pain) but might have anti-inflammatory properties in the leukocyte-mediated events of chronic inflammation, associated with tissue proliferation and 'repair' mechanisms [for review, see ref. 10].

Another aspect is the action of NSAID on the formation of other products of arachidonic acid peroxidation, namely hydroperoxy and hydroxy acids (HPETEs and HETEs) including leukotrienes, as well as oxygen-centered radicals (fig. 1). HPETEs and HETEs are major products of arachidonic acid metabolism in leukocytes and platelets and exhibit chemotactic properties for white cells [11]. It has been suggested that certain NSAID may inhibit the lipoxygenase pathways, preventing the formation of these products [5].

5-Benzoyl-α-methyl-2-thiophene-acetic acid (tiaprofenic acid) is a recently developed agent, capable of inhibition of prostaglandin formation and possessing potent anti-inflammatory activities in an animal model of inflammation [2]. We have studied the actions of this compound on vascular PGI_2 and platelet thromboxane formation and aggregation [6, 8]. In addition, we have investigated the effects of this compound on collagen-induced platelet aggregation and thromboxane formation after oral administration in humans. The present study also includes preliminary data on the inhibition of platelet lipoxygenase by this agent.

Materials and Methods

Generation and Measurement of PGI₂

Generation and Measurement of PGI$_2$

Subepicardial coronary arteries were prepared from fresh bovine hearts, cut into rings and equilibrated for at least 2–3 h in oxygenated Krebs-Henseleit (K-H) buffer. Rings (90–100 mg) were transferred into reaction vials, containing $500 \mu l$ K-H buffer at $37 °C$. PGI$_2$ formation was stimulated by adding arachidonic acid ($3 \mu mol/l$) for 4 min. The NSAID or the respective solvent were added 10 min prior to arachidonic acid to the vascular rings in the reaction vials. PGI$_2$-like activity was estimated by measuring the antiaggregatory effect of aliquots of the vessel incubates on ADP-induced primary aggregation of human platelets in platelet-rich plasma (PRP) as described in detail elsewhere [8]. Synthetic PGI$_2$-sodium (Dr. *Bartmann,* Hoechst, Frankfurt) was used as standard. The validity of this assay technique was established previously by measuring immunoreactive 6-oxo-PGF$_{1\alpha}$ in the same probes that were bioassayed for PGI$_2$ [7].

Platelet Aggregation Studies

Platelet Aggregation Studies

Venous blood was taken from volunteers, including the test persons (see below), and collected into acidic citrate dextrose (ACD) (12:1, v/v) (Biostabil®, Biotest, Frankfurt, FRG). None of these subjects had received any NSAID-containing medication during the previous week. PRP was prepared by centrifugation at $300 g$ at room temperature for 10 min. Platelet aggregation was studied in a two-channel aggregometer (Labor, Hamburg, FRG) by measuring the changes in light transmission. ADP (Boehringer, Mannheim, FRG) ($5–20 \mu g/ml$), arachidonic acid (Nu-Chek, Elysian, Minnesota) (0.2 mmol/l) and collagen (Horm-Chemie, München, FRG) ($0.3–10 \mu g/ml$) were used as aggregating agents. The NSAID or the respective solvent were added 10 min prior to the aggregating agent to the PRP in the in vitro studies [for more details, see ref. 8].

Generation and Measurement of Thromboxanes

Generation and Measurement of Thromboxanes

Platelets were separated from the PRP by centrifugation for 7.5 min at $1,750 g$, washed and resuspended in an isotonic sodium-phosphate buffer (pH 6.8), supplemented with glucose (5 mmol/l). The platelet count was adjusted to 2×10^8 platelets/ml (TOA Counter). Thromboxane formation was initiated by addition of arachidonic acid ($30 \mu mol/l$) or thrombin (Topostasin®, Hoffmann-La Roche, Basel) (0.6 IU/ml) to $400 \mu l$ of the platelet suspension. The incubation time was 30 s at $37 °C$. Thereafter, the incubate was immediately transferred into an organ bath containing a rabbit aorta strip for measuring 'rabbit aorta contracting substance' (RCS), an equivalent for TXA$_2$ as described in detail elsewhere [8]. The validity of this technique was established previously by measuring immunoreactive TXB$_2$ in the same probes that were used for bioassaying RCS [7]. The NSAID or the respective solvent were added 10 min prior to arachidonic acid or thrombin to the washed platelet suspensions.

Platelet Lipoxygenase

Platelet Lipoxygenase

Washed platelet suspensions were freeze-thawed three times in a dry ice-acetone bath. The cell debris was removed by high-speed centrifugation. The supernatant was decanted and the protein content assayed according to Lowry. The reaction medium contained: Tris buffer pH 8.0 (50 mmol/l), platelet cytoplasmic fraction equivalent to 2 mg protein, arachidonic acid (50 nmol) and the NSAID or the respective solvent in a total volume of 1 ml. The cytoplasmic fraction was incubated for 5 min at $37 °C$ with the NSAID or solvent before addition of arachidonic acid. The reaction product, 12-HPETE, was measured in a dual wavelength mode (Aminco DW 2, Colora, Lorch, FRG) at 240 nm by determining the linear protion of the initial slope, according to the techniques described by *Sun* et al. [9].

Oral Administration of Tiaprofenic Acid

6 healthy volunteers (4 male, 2 female) between the ages of 22 and 39 years participated in this study. Informed consent was obtained from all vounteers. Following a standard breakfast, 400 mg tiaprofenic acid were administered orally. Immediately prior to the administration (time 0) and 1, 2, 3. 4.5, 6 and 12 h thereafter, blood was taken by venipuncture, collected into ACD and used for preparation of PRP as described above. Another portion of the blood was allowed to aggregate. The serum was decanted and subjected to determination of tiaprofenic acid.

Substances

Tiaprofenic acid (Albert-Roussel, Wiesbaden, FRG), indomethacin (Merck, Sharp & Dohme, München, FRG) diclofenac sodium (Ciba-Geigy, Basel, Switzerland), meclofenamate (Warner-Lambert/Parke-Davis, Pontypool, UK), 5,8,11,14-eicosatetraynoic acid (ETYA) (Sandoz, Basel, Switzerland). ETYA was dissolved in absolute ethanol at 1 mg/ml, the other substances as described elsewhere [8]. These agents were kindly provided by the respective manufacturers.

Results

PGI_2 Formation

Incubation of bovine coronary artery rings with arachidonic acid (3 µmol/l) was followed by a dose- and time-dependent PGI_2 formation amounting to 10.5 ± 2.8 nmol/l PGI_2 within 4 min in the incubation medium. A 20-µl aliquot, equivalent to 0.42 nmol/l PGI_2 was found to give an about 40–50% inhibition of platelet aggregation and was used in the further studies. Treatment of the rings with NSAID, concentration-dependently inhibited the PGI_2 formation. Compared to indomethacin, diclofenac was slightly more ($p < 0.05$), tiaprofenic acid was slightly less ($p < 0.05$) potent (table I). A single experiment with tiaprofenic acid is demonstrated as figure 2.

Platelet Aggregation

None of the NSAID studied influenced the ADP-induced primary aggregation of PRP. However, there was a significant and dose-dependent inhibition of both the collagen- and arachidonic acid-induced aggregations (table II).

Thromboxane Formation

All of the agents studied produced a concentration-dependent inhibition of the arachidonic acid-induced TXA_2 (RCS) formation in washed human

Table I. Inhibition of vascular cyclooxygenase (PGI_2 formation)

Substance	50% inhibition of PGI_2 formation, μmol/ml	
	n	$\bar{x} \pm$ SEM
Indomethacin	6	0.6 ± 0.1[1]
Tiaprofenic acid	6	1.0 ± 0.1[1]
Diclofenac	6	0.4 ± 0.1[1]
Meclofenamate	8	0.6 ± 0.2

[1] Data from *Kuhn* et al. [6].

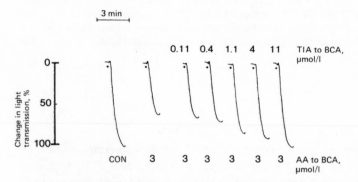

Fig. 2. Inhibition of release of antiaggregatory, PGI_2-like activity from bovine coronary artery (BCA) by tiaprofenic acid (TIA) in vitro. ● = Addition of ADP to the platelet-rich plasma, containing an aliquot of the arachidonic acid (AA) + BCA incubate; CON = control (PRP + ADP + tiaprofenic acid solvent).

Table II. Inhibition of platelet aggregation in vitro

Substance	50% inhibition of platelet aggregation, μmol/l			
	arachidonic acid-induced		collagen-induced	
	n	$\bar{x} \pm$ SEM	n	$\bar{x} \pm$ SEM
Indomethacin	7	0.5 ± 0.1	7	0.3 ± 0.1
Tiaprofenic acid	6	0.9 ± 0.2	7	3.8 ± 0.7
Diclofenac	6	0.4 ± 0.1	7	0.5 ± 0.1
Meclofenamate	5	0.8 ± 0.2	6	1.9 ± 0.2

Table III. Inhibition of platelet cyclooxygenase (thromboxane A_2 + HHT formation)

Substance	50% inhibition of «RCS» formation, µmol/l			
	arachidonic acid-induced		thrombin-induced	
	n	$\bar{x} \pm$ SEM	n	$\bar{x} \pm$ SEM
Indomethacin	48	0.019 ± 0.003^1	5	0.007 ± 0.001
Tiaprofenic acid	6	0.070 ± 0.024^1	9	0.021 ± 0.006
Diclofenac	12	63.0 ± 5.8^1	6	0.024 ± 0.009
Meclofenamate	6	45.0 ± 12.0^1	4	0.039 ± 0.004

[1] Data from *Schrör* et al. [8].

Table IV. Inhibition of platelet lipoxygenase (12-HPETE formation)

Substance	IC_{50}, µmol/l
ETYA	0.20
	0.16
	0.07
Indomethacin	> 28.0
	22.0
Tiaprofenic acid	153.0
	230.0
	> 153.0

platelets. Indomethacin and tiaprofenic acid were the most active compounds, whereas diclofenac and meclofenamate were 2–3 orders of magnitude less potent. Using thrombin as stimulating agent, the IC_{50} for indomethacin and tiaprofenic acid remained the same whereas that of meclofenamate and diclofenac were reduced to the level of tiaprofenic acid (table III).

Platelet Lipoxygenase

The formation of 12-HPETE was concentration-dependently inhibited by ETYA, the IC_{50} ranging between 0.07 and 0.20 µmol/l. The IC_{50} for indomethacin and tiaprofenic acid were 2–3 orders of magnitude higher (table IV).

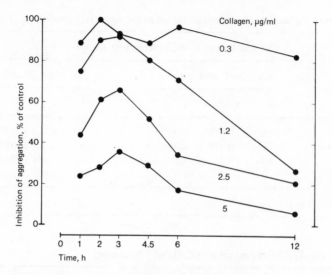

Fig. 3. Inhibition of collagen-induced platelet aggregation ex vivo after oral administration of tiaprofenic acid at time 0. The control aggregation before administration of the drug was set 0% inhibition. Each point represents the mean of 6 observations. Note the decrease in inhibition by enhancing the collagen concentration and the time dependency of this response.

Oral Administration of Tiaprofenic Acid

No side effects were reported by any of the subjects tested. The serum concentration of tiaprofenic acid reached a maximum after 2 h, equivalent to $125 \pm 25 \mu mol/l$ and was reduced to $60 \mu mol/l$ at 4.5 h. The platelet count in the PRP was $607 \pm 95 \times 10^3/\mu l$ at time 0, $647 \pm 116 \times 10^3/\mu l$ at 2 h and $589 \pm 80 \times 10^3/\mu l$ at 6 h after oral administration ($p > 0.05$). Ex vivo, there was no change in the ADP-induced primary aggregation of platelets at any time of the study. In contrast, a time-dependent inhibition of collagen-induced aggregation was apparent which was antagonized by increasing the collagen concentration (fig. 3). An original recording together with the measured serum concentration of tiaprofenic acid in this subject is demonstrated in figure 4.

The arachidonic acid-induced aggregation was completely suppressed in 3 out of 3 subjects studied at time 1 h and remained inhibited up to 6 h.

Discussion

Present data indicate that tiaprofenic acid is a potent cyclooxygenase inhibiting agent in vitro. This became evident in particular from the studies

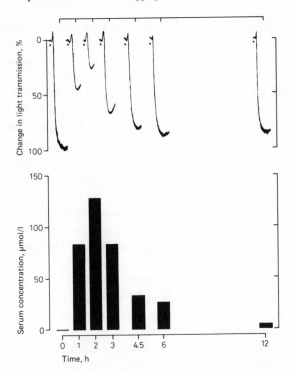

Fig. 4. Changes in collagen-induced (2.5 µg/ml) platelet aggregation ex vivo and serum level of tiaprofenic acid after oral administration of 400 mg tiaprofenic acid to 1 human volunteer (22 years, male). Tiaprofenic acid was given immediately after taking the control reading at time 0.

on RCS formation of washed human platelets. The concentration, required for a 50% inhibition of RCS release (IC_{50}) after addition of arachidonic acid was 70 nmol/l and in the same range as indomethacin but 2–3 orders of magnitude lower than that for the two fenamates studied. Using thrombin as stimulus for RCS formation, these differences apparently disappeared. This suggests that fenamates might have additional effects on thrombin-induced events of platelet activation, such as liberation of endogenous arachidonic acid, which are not involved in the actions of tiaprofenic acid and indomethacin at the concentrations used.

The thromboxane synthetase of human platelets also catalyses the formation of HHT [3], a chemotactic compound for white cells [4]. Thus, reduction of the PG endoperoxides in the platelet by inhibition of the cyclooxygenase will also inhibit the HHT formation. There is histopathological evidence for platelet activation and coagulation in the microcirculation in inflamed areas [for review, see ref. 10]. Inhibition of formation of these cyclooxygenase-derived products might be clinically important for the mode of action of these drugs.

As expected, all NSAID studied antagonized the arachidonic- and collagen-induced aggregation of human platelets in PRP in vitro but did not modify the primary ADP-induced aggregation. The IC_{50} for both kinds of stimulation was between 0.3 and 3.8 μmol/l and in the same range as previous studies with rabbit PRP [6]. By comparing the arachidonic acid-induced aggregation with RCS release, it is evident that both tiaprofenic acid and indomethacin inhibit the RCS formation at significantly lower concentrations than required for inhibition of platelet aggregation. This might be due to the absence of plasma in the washed platelet suspensions, because more than 90% of these compounds is bound to plasma albumin. However, the same consideration can also be applied to the fenamates and no such difference in inhibition of platelet aggregation between these agents and tiaprofenic acid was seen. It has been suggested that platelet aggregation and activation of the arachidonic acid pathway in platelets might not be tightly coupled. This would agree with our data.

Oral administration of tiaprofenic acid was found to inhibit the collagen- and arachidonic acid-induced aggregation ex vivo. This inhibition was a transient response and apparently correlated to the serum levels of the compound. Interestingly, more than 100 μmol/l serum tiaprofenic acid were needed to obtain a 50% inhibition of collagen (1.25 μg/ml)-induced platelet aggregation ex vivo and this response was considerably attenuated by increasing the collagen concentration up to 5 μg/ml. In contrast, a 50% inhibition of collagen-induced aggregation by tiaprofenic acid in vitro was achieved at 4 μmol/l at the same or even higher collagen concentrations. We do not yet have a sufficient explanation for this apparent difference. It could be that due to the limited protein content in vitro the amount of bound tiaprofenic acid is reduced and more substance available in the unbound and biologically active form. Alternatively, long-time incubation of platelets with tiaprofenic acid in vivo might produce changes in the platelet reactivity which makes them less sensitive against aggregating agents.

Inhibition of the coronary vascular cyclooxygenase and consecutive PGI_2 formation required higher amounts of tiaprofenic acid and indomethacin than the inhibition of the platelet cyclooxygenase and consecutive TX and HHT formation. Both studies have been carried out in plasma-free media in vitro. Therefore, no direct conclusions can be drawn to the in vivo situation, also, because the cyclooxygenases were derived from tissues of different species. However, the large differences in concentrations of tiaprofenic acid and indomethacin, required to inhibit the arachidonic acid-induced TX formation and arachidonic acid-induced PGI_2 formation might indicate a 'split' between vascular and platelets' cyclooxygenases, which one should look into more in detail.

In conclusion, our data suggest that tiaprofenic acid is a cyclooxygenase-inhibiting agent that is particularly effective against the platelet enzyme and probably does not inactivate the platelet lipoxygenase. To what extent this mechanism of action is involved in the anti-inflammatory properties of this agent in vivo [2], cannot be answered by these in vitro data. However, the low inhibitory potential of the substance on vascular PGI_2 formation associated with a rapid recovery within a few minutes in vitro might be therapeutically important and should be studied further.

References

1   Burch, J.W.; Stanford, N.; Majerus, P.W.: Inhibition of platelet prostaglandin synthetase by oral aspirin. J. clin. Invest. *61:* 314–319 (1978).

2   Deraedt, R.; Jouquey, S.; Delevallee, F.; Flahaut, M.: Release of prostaglandins E and F in algogenic reactions and its inhibition. Eur. J. Pharmacol. *61:* 17–24 (1980).

3   Diczfalusy, U.; Hammarström, S.: Conversion of prostaglandin endoperoxides to C_{17}-hydroxy acids catalyzed by human platelet thromboxane synthetase. FEBS Lett. *84:* 271–274 (1977).

4   Goetzl, E.J.; Gorman, R.R.: Chemotactic and chemokinetic stimulation of human eosinophil and neutrophil polymorphonuclear leukocytes by 12-L-hydroxy-5,8,10-heptadecatrienoic acid (HHT). J. Immun. *120:* 526–531 (1978).

5   Higgs, G.A.; Flower, R.J.; Vane, J.R.: A new approach to antiinflammatory drugs. Biochem. Pharmac. *28:* 1959–1961 (1979).

6   Kuhn, A.; Sauerland, S.; Schiffer, K.; Schrör, K.: The action of non-steroidal antiinflammatory agents on platelet aggregation and vessel tone in relation to inhibition of PGI_2 and thromboxane release. With particular reference to 5-benzoyl-α-methyl-2-thiophene acetic acid (tiaprofenic acid). Arzneimittel-Forsch. *30:* 1538–1542 (1980).

7   Schrör, K.; Köhler, P.; Müller, M.; Peskar, B.A.; Rösen, P.: Prostacyclin-thromboxane interactions in the platelet-perfused in vitro heart. Am. J. Physiol. *241:* H18–H25 (1981).

8   Schrör, K.; Sauerland, S.; Kuhn, A.; Rösen, R.: Different sensitivities of prostaglandin cyclooxygenases in blood platelets and coronary arteries against non-steroidal antiinflammatory drugs. Arch. Pharmacol. *313:* 69–76 (1980).

9   Sun, F.F.; McGuire, J.C.; Morton, D.R.; Pike, J.E.; Sprecher, H.; Kunau, W.H.: Inhibition of platelet arachidonic acid 12-lipoxygenase by acetylenic acid compounds. Prostaglandins *21:* 333–343 (1981).

10 Trang, L.E.: Prostaglandins and inflammation. Semin. Arthrit. Rheumatism *9:* 153–190 (1980).
11 Turner, S.R.; Tainer, J.A.; Lynn, W.S.: Biogenesis of chemotactic molecules by the arachidonate lipoxygenase system of blood platelets. Nature, Lond. *257:* 680–681 (1975).
12 Vane, J.R.: Inhibition of prostaglandin synthesis as a mechanism of action for aspirin-like drugs. Nature new Biol. *231:* 232–235 (1971).
13 Whittle, B.J.R.: Selective inhibition of prostaglandin production in inflammatory exsudates and gastric mucosa. Nature, Lond. *284:* 271–273 (1980).

K. Schrör, MD, Pharmakologisches Institut der Universität Köln, Gleueler Strasse 24, D-5000 Köln 41 (FRG)

Rheumatology, vol. 7, pp. 99–106 (Karger, Basel 1982)

Pharmacokinetic Interaction between Tiaprofenic Acid and Several Other Compounds for Chronic Use

P.W. Lücker[a], B. Penth[b], K. Wetzelsberger[a]

[a]Institut für klinische Pharmakologie, Bobenheim/Berg, BRD; [b]Albert-Roussel Pharma GmbH, Wiesbaden, BRD

Introduction

Nonsteroidal antirheumatics have a high clinical impact in the treatment of rheumatic diseases especially in osteoarthritis. The advantages of nonsteroidal antirheumatics are obvious and are not a matter of discussion here. The problems arising concerning continuous treatment of chronic diseases are the pharmacokinetic interactions of drugs that could be administered simultaneously and for a long period of time.

Tiaprofenic acid is a new approach to treat rheumatoid diseases and for this reason we investigated the pharmacokinetics of tiaprofenic acid as well as the dynamic and kinetic interaction with some other commonly used drugs.

A literature search gave us some excellent information about the pharmacokinetics of tiaprofenic acid in humans, issued by *Pottier* et al. [2]. The authors used a ^{14}C-labelled compound and clarified the pharmacokinetic model as well as the parameters. All their results could be proved later on by our group using a chemical method [1].

To establish the pharmacokinetic profile of tiaprofenic acid, we first ran a study on 7 healthy subjects after having developed a method for the determination of tiaprofenic acid in human serum. In a second study the pharmacokinetic interaction with $Al(OH)_3$ and ASA was investigated. In a third study tiaprofenic acid was administered after pretreatment with phenprocoumon.

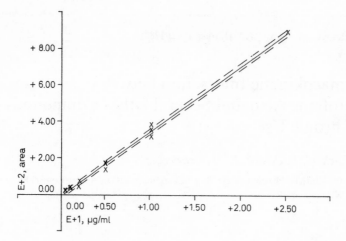

Fig. 1. Standard curve of tiaprofenic acid in serum. Linearity is proved by the regression.

Material and Methods

Assay of Tiaprofenic Acid

0.35 mmol/l hydrochloric acid was added to the serum and then extracted three times in diethylether. The three extracts are combined and totally dried with a rotatory evaporator. The residuals are solved again in methanol and injected onto an HPLC column. The measurements were performed at a wavelength of 308 nm on an HPLC device (Hewlett Packard 1084 B). The variance of the method amounted to 4.89%. The standard curve was linear down to 500 ng/ml (fig. 1). The method was appropriate for the pharmacokinetic analysis [1].

Assay of Phenprocoumon

After acidic extraction with chloroform from serum, pH ist detected after HPLC separation at 315 nm. The calibration curve is linear between 0.1 and 5 µg/ml.

Subjects

For the different studies we had several groups of healthy male subjects at our disposal that gave written consent after having been informed about the risks and the aim of the study. To obtain good pharmacokinetic results with a minimum of variation the volunteers were hospitalized 36 h before the administration of the drug. They were put on a light diet and they had to drink 2 liters of water the day before administration. After the administration, together with a standard breakfast, the subjects fasted for 8 h. The blood was sampled for up to 24 h after the administration.

First Study

One of the volunteers received 600 mg tiaprofenic acid and 6 of them received 200 mg in the course of the pharmacokinetic study. In the second part of the study the subjects received Al(OH)$_3$ and ASA together with 200 mg of tiaprofenic acid.

Second Study
In the second study pentoxyphylline and 200 mg of tiaprofenic acid was administered.

Third Study
The third study was designed to find out the effect of tiaprofenic acid on PTT and Quick values after a pretreatment with phenprocoumon and the pharmacokinetic interaction of phenprocoumon and tiaprofenic acid.

Results

Pharmacokinetics
The pharmacokinetics of tiaprofenic acid are linear. A saturation process could not be detected:

$$\frac{AUC_o\ 600\ mg}{AUC_o\ 400\ mg} = \frac{110.9}{73.1}$$

$$\frac{73.1 \cdot 600}{43.8} = \frac{400 \cdot 110.9}{44.3}$$

It can be seen that there is no influence on the bioavailability caused by different dosages between 400 and 600 mg of tiaprofenic acid.

The pharmacokinetic profile of tiaprofenic acid showed 2 peaks at 1.2 and 2.9 h in 3 of the volunteers, so that we calculated the pharmacokinetic parameters model-free (fig. 2). Three other subjects showed curves with 1 peak (fig. 3), the parameters of these volunteers were calculated by curve-fitting to an open one-compartment model.

The mean biological half-life was calculated from the second curve in group 1 and the elimination process of the group 2 and amounted to 1.1 h. The mean area under the curve taking both curves of group 1 into consideration amounted to 73.1 µg/h/ml. The total clearance was calculated as 6 liters/h. The central volume of distribution was 8.6 liters. This gives a hint that tiaprofenic acid is not distributed in the body water. The peak of concentration in the urine was reached after 2 h.

The renal excretion of the compound is finished after roughly 12 h, which is in good accordance with the biological half-life (fig. 4).

The half-life could also be proved by the renal excretion of the drug. Tiaprofenic acid is partly cleared by the kidneys, the renal clearance amounts to 0.3 liters/h, i.e. 5% (fig. 5).

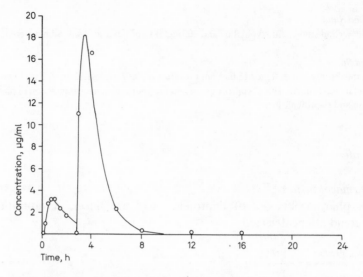

Fig. 2. Typical profile of tiaprofenic acid as found in 3 of 7 subjects, probably caused by the simultaneously administered standard breakfast.

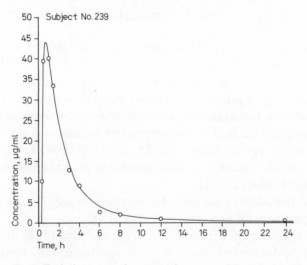

Fig. 3. Typical concentration versus time curve of tiaprofenic acid.

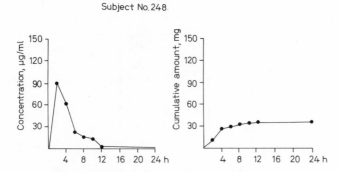

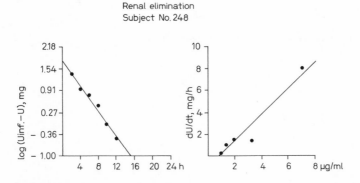

Fig. 4. Urinary concentration versus time plot (left curve). The cumulative excretion is plotted on the right curve.

Fig. 5. Graphic half-life determination (left curve) and renal clearance (right curve).

Interactions

After the pharmacokinetics of tiaprofenic acid were established we checked the pharmacokinetic interaction with several other drugs. Figure 6 shows that there is no major influence on the pharmacokinetics of tiaprofenic acid when aluminium hydroxide, acetyl-salicylic acid, pentoxyphylline or phenprocoumon is administered at the same time, as far as the bioavailability is concerned. The analysis of variance was used for statistical analysis.

For clinical use, it is important to have information about the transit time. The transit time [4] is the mean time one molecule of tiaprofenic acid needs to pass the organism and give information of time dependency of the LADME system (fig. 7).

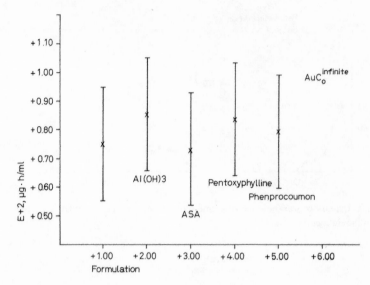

Fig. 6. Column means of the AUCs of different studies.

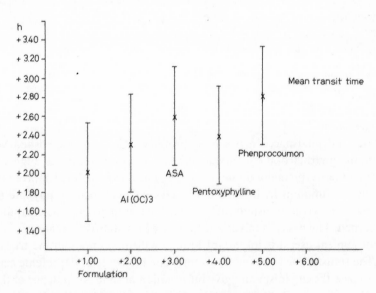

Fig. 7. Column means of the transit time of different studies.

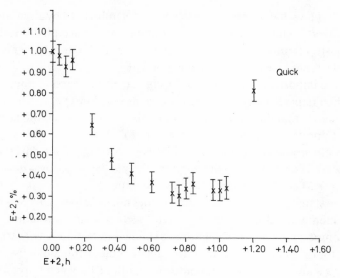

Fig. 8. Column means of the Quick values during the study.

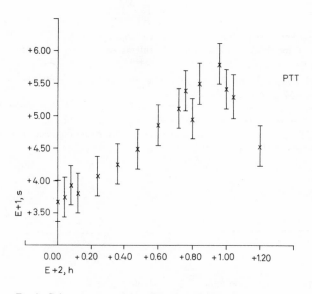

Fig. 9. Column means of the PTT values during the study.

Figure 7 shows that the mean transit time is not influenced by aluminium hydroxide, acetyl salicylic acid, phenprocoumon, or pentoxyphylline. The simultaneously administered phenprocoumon showed a slightly longer transit time that cannot be explained for the moment.

It seemed important to us to check the clinical effectiveness of phenprocoumon when tiaprofenic acid is administered at very low Quick values [3]. It could be shown that there is no influence on the blood coagulation parameters when tiaprofenic acid is administered (fig. 8).

The administration of tiaprofenic acid was given on day 7 and day 9. The Quick values did not change. On the evening of day 9, the subject was injected with vitamin K. The Quick values increased as expected.

It can be stated that the dosage regimen does not have to be altered when one of the mentioned drugs is administered together with tiaprofenic acid. The new compound is, as far as pharmacokinetic interaction is concerned, a safe drug for use in the daily medical treatment of the rheumatoid diseases.

Figure 9 shows that there is no influence on the PTT when tiaprofenic acid is administered at high PTT levels. Tiaprofenic acid was given on days 7 and 9. The PTT values did not change. The subjects were injected with vitamin K on the evening of day 9. The PTT decreased as expected.

References

1   Maracek, N.; Lücker, P.W.; Altmayer, P.; Wetzelsberger, K.; Penth, B.: Zur Pharmakokinetik von Tiaprofensäure und zur Frage der Interaktion mit ASS und Aluminiumhydroxid. Arzneimittel-Forsch. *31:* 116–120 (1981).

2   Pottier, J.; Cousty-Berlin, D.; Busigny, M.: Human pharmacokinetics of tiaprofenic acid. Reports AG 12, AD 54, AF 11, AD 95, and AF 58.

3   Dürr, J.; Pfeiffer, M.H.; Penth, B.; Wetzelsberger, K.; Lücker, P.W.: Untersuchung zur Frage einer Interaktion von Tiaprofensäure und Phenprocoumon (in press).

4   Hattingberg, H.M. von; Brockmeier, D.: The pharmacokinetic basis of optimal antibiotic dosage. Infection *8:* 21–24 (1980).

Prof. Dr. P.W. Lücker, Institut für klinische Pharmakologie,
D-6719 Bobenheim am Berg (FRG)

Rheumatology, vol. 7, pp. 107–110 (Karger, Basel 1982)

A Comparison of Gastrointestinal Bleeding in Healthy Volunteers Treated with Tiaprofenic Acid, Aspirin or Ibuprofen

S.J. Warrington, A. Halsey, L. O'Donnell

Charterhouse Clinical Research Unit Limited, London, England

Introduction

Aspirin is an effective anti-inflammatory drug but, in chronic use, it is associated with a high incidence of gastrointestinal side effects including acute and chronic blood loss [1, 2, 4, 7]. Newer agents, such as ibuprofen, are less likely to cause gastric disturbance and bleeding [4–6]. Tiaprofenic acid is an effective anti-inflammatory drug but its effect on gastrointestinal blood loss in man has not previously been fully investigated. This study compared faecal blood loss in healthy men receiving aspirin, ibuprofen or tiaprofenic acid, using a double-blind, parallel group design.

Subjects and Methods

The subjects were 30 healthy men with regular bowel habits aged 19–26 years and weighing 63–95 kg. They were asked to abstain from alcoholic drinks and breakfast cereals for the duration of the study. Routine laboratory tests were carried out before and at the end of the study. Subjects with a history of significant disease, peptic ulcer or gastric intolerance, or known to be sensitive to aspirin or propionic acid derivatives were excluded. No concurrent medication was allowed.

After an initial week on placebo, the subjects were randomly allocated to one of the three treatment groups for 2 weeks: (1) tiaprofenic acid 200 mg thrice daily; (2) ibuprofen 400 mg thrice daily, or (3) aspirin 600 mg thrice daily.

On the first day of placebo treatment, 10 ml of venous blood from each subject was labelled with 50μCi ^{51}Cr as sodium chromate, using standard methods [3], and re-injected. All stools passed were then collected daily until 2 days after the end of medication. In order to identify the first stool sample in which blood content could have been influenced by the trial drugs, each subject ingested 1μCi ^{58}Co (4 subjects) or ^{57}Co (26 subjects) as cobaltous chloride dissolved in

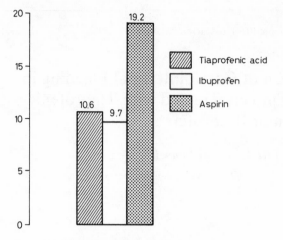

Fig. 1. Total blood loss (days 12–23).

water, at the start of active treatment; this substance is virtually nonabsorbed during its passage through the gut.

The ^{51}Cr in each sample was measured using a whole body counter and compared with a ^{51}Cr standard solution. The ^{57}Co or ^{58}Co activity was separately displayed by a multichannel analyser. The volume of blood in each sample was estimated from the faecal ^{51}Cr content after correction for decay, the injected dose of ^{51}Cr, and subjects' blood volume derived from a nomogram; this method consistently underestimates faecal blood loss because it ignores urinary excretion of ^{51}Cr not bound to red cells.

For blood loss calculations, the 'trial period' was taken as day 1 to the day before the appearance of the cobaltous tracer dose in the stools and the 'treatment period' was taken from day 12 to day 23, that is, until 2 days after the end of active treatment. Where a subject had no bowel motion on a particular day, the blood loss for that day was estimated by apportioning the loss in the next stool collection equally between the stool-free days. Comparisons of the blood losses for the three treatment groups were made by nonparametric methods (Kruskal-Wallis test).

Results

All three treatments were well tolerated clinically and no subject noticed overt blood loss. There were no changes in any of the laboratory tests. Total blood loss during the treatment period with tiaprofenic acid was 10.6 ml, with ibuprofen 9.7 ml and with aspirin 19.2 ml. The loss was significantly higher in the aspirin group ($p < 0.05$) (fig. 1). Mean daily blood loss was significantly higher on all three drugs than on placebo ($p < 0.05$). The increase in blood

Table I. Mean daily blood loss

	Tiaprofenic acid group		Ibuprofen group		Aspirin group	
	active	placebo	active	placebo	active	placebo
Mean daily blood loss, ml	0.88	0.25	0.81	0.26	1.6	0.31
Increase in mean daily blood loss during active treatment, ml	0.63		0.55		1.29	

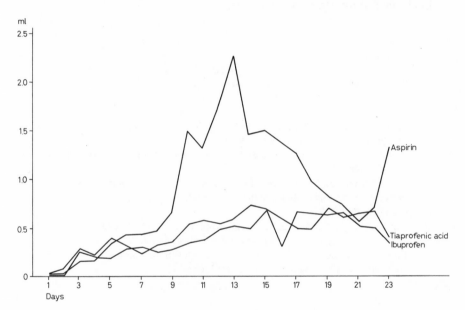

Fig. 2. Median daily blood loss per group.

loss during aspirin administration was significantly greater than the increase in blood loss during ibuprofen treatment ($p < 0.05$) and approached significance when compared to the increase in blood loss during tiaprofenic acid treatment ($0.05 < p < 0.1$) (table I). The median daily blood loss for the three groups is shown in figure 2. Two subjects, 1 taking tiaprofenic acid and the other ibuprofen, showed transient but substantial increases in faecal blood loss during treatment, against a background of otherwise low losses. Both subjects remained asymptomatic and they denied alcohol abuse during the study.

Discussion

All three anti-inflammatory drugs increased gastrointestinal blood loss but aspirin caused significantly greater losses than the other two treatments. There was no significant difference between the results for tiaprofenic acid and ibuprofen. Since ibuprofen is generally very well tolerated in clinical practice, these results suggest that tiaprofenic acid may be similarly free from the propensity to cause gastrointestinal bleeding. Nevertheless, the safety of any new drug should evidently be confirmed by careful observation during its chronic administration to patients.

References

1   Benson, T.A.: Gastrointestinal reactions to drugs. Am. J. dig. Dis. *16:* 357–362 (1971).
2   Croft, D.-N.; Wood, P.H.N.: Gastric mucosa and susceptibility to occult gastrointestinal bleeding caused by aspirin. Br. med. J. *i:* 137–141 (1967).
3   Davies, J.W.: Blood volume studies; in Belcher, Vetter, Radioistopes in medical diagnosis, pp. 319–341 (Butterworths, London 1971).
4   Dick, W.C.; Buchanan, W.: Advances in the treatment of rheumatic disorders. Practitioner *207:* 483–491 (1971).
5   Hall, J.E.; Agar, J.; Buckler, J.W.; Dodsworth, P.G.; Goldberg, A.A.J.: Ibuprofen in the treatment of rheumatic diseases with particular reference to long-term therapy. Therapie-woche *37:* 3293 (1973).
6   Lanza, F.; Royer, G.; Nelson, R.: An endoscopic evaluation of the effects of non-steroidal anti-inflammatory drugs on the gastric mucosa. Gastrointest. Endosc. *21:* 103 (1975).
7   Leonards, J.R.; Levy, G.: Gastrointestinal blood loss from aspirin and sodium salicylate tablets in man. Clin. Pharmacol. Ther. *14:* 62–66 (1973).

S.J. Warrington, MD, Charterhouse Clinical Research Unit Limited, Boundary House, 91/93 Charterhouse Street, London EC 1 (England)

Rheumatology, vol. 7, pp. 111–117 (Karger, Basel 1982)

Interaction of Tiaprofenic Acid and Acenocoumarol

J. Meurice

'Le Valdor' Gerontological Centre, Liège, Belgium

Introduction

Most nonsteroidal anti-inflammatory drugs potentiate the action of coumarin derivatives through displacement from their plasma protein-binding sites. In addition, some of them, e.g. aspirin, decrease prothrombin and proconvertin plasma concentrations even in the absence of a coumarin derivative. Since these drugs also have an ulcerogenic action, it is usually advised to be very cautious when prescribing them in association with an anticoagulant. In rats, tiaprofenic acid has no anticoagulant effect when administered alone at a dose of 25 mg/day for 9 days. However, when the same dose is given during the same amount of time with warfarin, it potentiates the anticoagulant effect of the latter. In animals pretreated for 7 days with the anticoagulant, and then treated for 2 days with tiaprofenic acid there is potentiation at a dose of 50 mg/kg. It was therefore thought necessary to study the clinical and biological tolerance of tiaprofenic acid in patients treated with a coumarin derivative.

Patients and Methods

Protocol

This open study was performed according to the following protocol which is summarized in figure 1.

Patient Inclusion. The patients included were 10 hospitalized patients of either sex, under anticoagulant therapy with a coumarin derivative, with stable coagulation factors and with a condition requiring treatment with an anti-inflammatory agent. Patients with a prothrombin time lower than 15% and patients with a history of hemorrhage were excluded.

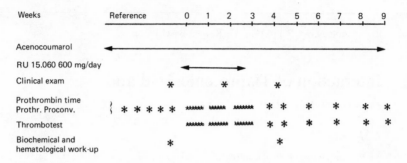

Fig. 1. Summary of the protocol. RU 15.060 = tiaprofenic acid.

Treatments. The anticoagulant treatment was acenocoumarol in 9 cases and phenprocoumon in 1 case; it was stabilized before the onset of the study and the dosage was not modified
during the study. Tiaprofenic acid was given as a one 200-mg tablet three times a day for at least
2 weeks. Concomitant medications were allowed as long as they did not affect coagulation.

Evaluation Criteria. Prothrombin time and prothrombin-proconvertin concentration were
measured several times during the reference period, six times a week during the tiaprofenic acid
treatment and several times at a decreasing rate during 6–8 weeks following discontinuation of
treatment. Owren's thrombotest was also measured during the latter two periods. Clinical examinations were performed and recorded before, during, and after tiaprofenic acid treatment.

The following biochemical and hematogical data were obtained before and after treatment: blood glucose, uric acid, creatinine, urea, SGOT, SGPT, alkaline phosphatase, sodium,
potassium, chlorine, total plasma proteins, albumin and hemoglobin, hematocrit, red and white
blood cell counts, differential and platelets.

Statistical Analysis

For each patient, each coagulation test and each period (before, during and after treatment
with tiaprofenic acid) a regression line was fitted through the observed points and compared to
the horizontal in order to see whether there was a tendency for the values to increase or decrease
with time during that period. For each patient and each of the three coagulation tests the means
of each of the three periods were compared through one-way analysis of variance and simple
contrasts if there was an overall significant difference. Mean values for the 10 patients were
obtained in the following way: (1) for the reference period (before treatment), one value representing the mean of the 10 individual means of all values of that test obtained during the reference period; (2) for the tiaprofenic acid treatment period, 15 values representing the means
across the 10 patients, of the first 15 treatment values obtained in each patient; (3) for the post-
treatment period, one mean value was computed for each week. A two-factor-analysis of
variance (patient × period) was used to compare the mean, the lowest and the highest value for
each period.

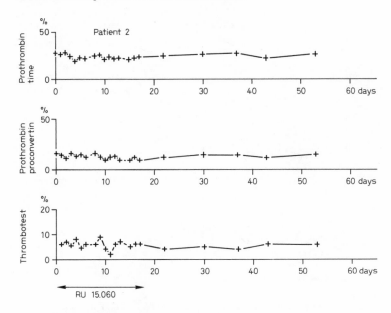

Fig. 2. Type of patient without modification. RU 15.060 = tiaprofenic acid.

Results

Patients' Characteristics

6 women and 4 men took part in the study. Their mean age was 66.2 years (SD 13.7 years) and 4 were older than 75 years. Their mean weight was 66.7 kg (SD 13.3 kg). 5 patients had had a cerebrovascular accident, 4 a myocardial infarct, and 1 patient had aortic stenosis. The anticoagulant drug was acenocoumarol in 9 patients and phenprocoumon in 1; the dose ranged from 1 to 8 mg/day and had been stable for at least 1 month, except in 3 patients where it had only been stable for 4–9 days. All patients had been on continuous antivitamin K therapy for at least 1 year except the last patient for whom the anticoagulant had been stopped and restarted 1 month before the study. In 5 patients, the reference period lasted several weeks. In 5 others, it lasted between 8 and 17 days. During that period, the mean prothrombin time ranged from $19.1 \pm 0.75\%$ (SEM) to $30.6 \pm 1.21\%$ and the mean prothrombin proconvertin level ranged from $14.4 \pm 1.47\%$ to $21.5 \pm 1.25\%$.

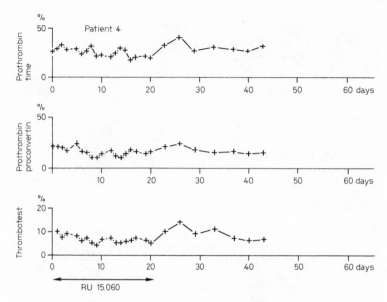

Fig. 3. Type of patient with rebound effect. RU 15.060 = tiaprofenic acid.

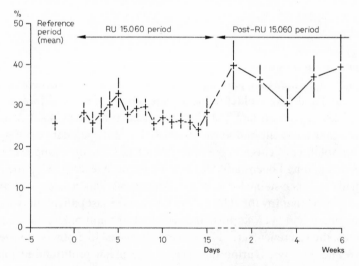

Fig. 4. Prothrombin time: mean values of 10 patients ± SEM. RU 15.060 = tiaprofenic acid.

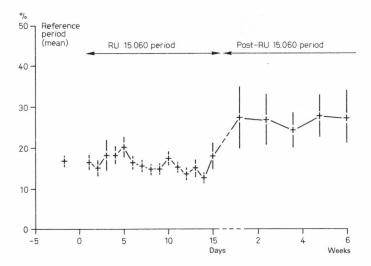

Fig. 5. Prothrombin-proconvertin: mean values of 10 patients ± SEM. RU 15.060 = tiaprofenic acid.

Evolution of Coagulation Parameters

Correlations between the three tests were good. There was a statistically significant tendency for both the prothrombin time and the prothrombin proconvertin level to increase in 2 patients and to decrease in 2 patients during the tiaprofenic acid period, whereas they had remained stable in all during the reference period. The modifications were moderate (± 10%). An example of the evolution of the three parameters during the study is shown in figure 2. Five patients behaved as this patient (patient 2). The other 5 patients behaved as patient 4 (shown in figure 3) in whom coagulation parameters increased immediately after discontinuation of tiaprofenic acid and came back to previous levels 1–3 weeks later.

For the latter patients the means of values obtained during the post-treatment period were significantly higher than the means of values obtained during the reference period and the tiaprofenic acid treatment period. This is reflected in figures 4–6, which show the evolution of the mean values for each of the three parameters: during tiaprofenic acid treatment, the mean values are the same as before treatment; after discontinuation of treatment the mean values are higher and the standard errors of these values greater. Plasma fibrinogen was measured in 4 patients several times during and after tiaprofenic acid. There was no significant variation.

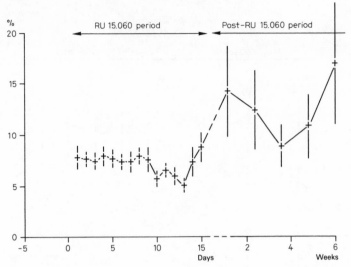

Fig. 6. Thrombotest: mean values of 10 patients ± SEM. RU 15.060 = tiaprofenic acid.

Clinical Examination and Biological Tolerance

There was no complaint and no change in physical examination. All blood values obtained were within normal ranges.

Discussion

Protocol

Among the 4 men and 6 women who took part in this study, 4 women were 80 or 81 years old, which is older than what had been planned initially. All patients had been on anticoagulants for over 1 year; for several patients, however, there had been a recent dosage modification, as recent as 6 days before the onset of the study.

Coagulation Tests

The trend analysis showed that prothrombin-proconvertin levels and prothrombin time were stabilized before the onset of treatment. It should be noted, however, that in 4 subjects the reference period lasted only 8–10 days and that in 2 additional subjects stabilization was obtained through a change in dosage. During tiaprofenic acid treatment, there was a tendency for the prothrombin time and the prothrombin-proconvertin level to increase in 2 subjects and a tendency to decrease in 2 other subjects. In the latter, the lowest value reached by the prothrombin time was 13% and changes were not greater than 10%. These moderate variations in both directions may be due to spontaneous evolution rather than an effect of tiaprofenic acid treatment.

Comparisons of mean, and of maximal and minimal values reached during each of the three periods showed no significant difference between the reference period and the tiaprofenic acid treatment period and significantly higher values during the post-treatment period. There was a large intersubject variation in this period, and 4 subjects demonstrated a marked rebound effect after discontinuation of tiaprofenic acid treatment. Three of these subjects were over 80 years of age, 2 of them had had a very short reference period, and 2 had had a recent modification of the anticoagulant dosage. For these subjects it would seem that tiaprofenic acid contributed to maintain coagulation tests within the desired range and that stopping it induced a rise in these parameters.

Conclusion

In this study, there was an interaction between tiaprofenic acid and acenocoumarol, as with most nonsteroidal anti-inflammatory drugs. It was not very obvious during at least 2 weeks of treatment with tiaprofenic acid, but became manifest after discontinuation of the drug in several patients. Modification of coagulation parameters was minimal in patients whose anticoagulant treatment had been stable for several months but greater in older patients or in patients whose antivitamin K dosage had been recently changed. When prescribing tiaprofenic acid to patients on antivitamin K treatment, it is, therefore, necessary to monitor the prothrombin time regularly during and after anti-inflammatory treatment, especially in older patients and in patients in whom the anticoagulant treatment is not perfectly stable.

J. Meurice, MD, Gerontological Centre, 'Le Valdor', 145 rue Basse-Wez, B-4020 Liège (Belgium)

Rheumatology, vol. 7, pp. 118–124 (Karger, Basel 1982)

A Dose-Ranging Study of Tiaprofenic Acid in Osteoarthritis

H. Berry, B. Bloom, E.B.D. Hamilton[1]

Department of Rheumatology, King's College Hospital, London, England

Introduction

Tiaprofenic acid (Surgam; α-(5-benzoyl-2-thienyl)-propionic acid) is a nonsteroidal anti-inflammatory agent of the thiophene group [2]. Clinical studies have shown 600 mg daily to be an effective dose in the treatment of osteoarthritis [3, 4, 6]. This study was designed to see whether 1.2 g daily tiaprofenic acid was more effective than 600 mg/day and to compare short-term tolerance.

Patients and Methods

A double-blind 3-way crossover study was carried out of 6 weeks duration, each patient receiving each treatment for 2 weeks, according to a randomised design. All six possible treatment orders were used. Prior to entry into the study all patients had a minimum 2-day washout period with access to paracetamol except those patients who had been taking a compound with a long carry-over effect, such as piroxicam, where the minimum washout period was 5 days. Patients included in the study were of either sex, aged 18 or more and suffering from osteoarthritis of the hip or knee confirmed by radiological features. They were all attending the hospital outpatient department. Pregnant women, patients with active peptic ulceration, severe hepatic or renal disease or those undergoing physiotherapy were excluded, as were patients on anticoagulants, immunosuppressives or oral hypoglycaemics or those known to be hypersensitive to propionic acid derivatives. Treatment consisted of double-blind tiaprofenic acid 600 mg daily, tiaprofenic acid 1.2 g daily and placebo, each patient receiving two tablets three times a day for each treatment. 84 paracetamol tablets were issued as a rescue analgesic for each treatment period. No other anti-inflammatory drug was allowed during the study.

[1] We are grateful to Dr. *K. MacRae* for the statistical analysis of this study, and to Miss *E.J. Thornton* of Roussel Laboratories for help in setting up and monitoring this study.

Patients were assessed on entry and at the end of each treatment period by the following parameters: pain on movement, night pain and pain at rest using both visual analogue scales, as described by *Berry and Huskisson* [1], and a four-point scale (none, mild, moderate or severe); duration (min) of morning stiffness; consumption of rescue analgesic; and patient preference. In addition, the number of trial tablets taken were recorded and drug assay of blood samples carried out at the end of each treatment period using HPLC [5]. Side effects were elicited by a simple non-leading question: 'Have the tablets upset you in any way?' Routine laboratory tests, including WBC, RBC, Hb, platelets, ESR, bilirubin, alkaline phosphatase, SGOT, γ-GT, urea and electrolytes, were also performed at each visit.

Results were analysed, using a parametric test (paired t test) and/or a non-parametric test (Wilcoxon's matched pairs signed ranks test) which were used to compare any two treatments. In most cases the same result regarding statistical significance was reached. However, in assessing the clinical results of treatment only the nonparametric tests result was used as such tests make fewer assumptions regarding the nature of the underlying statistical distributions. Because of missing values the number of patients in any comparison was sometimes less than 24. This was mainly where laboratory tests were concerned due to clotted samples.

Results

Of the original 24 patients entering the study two were found to be unsuitable and withdrawn very early on. One due to an unrelated abnormal initial laboratory test and one because the patient was found to be having treatment which should have exluded her from the study. Both these patients were replaced.

The mean age of the 24 patients analysed was 64 years, the mean weight 69.9 kg, the mean disease duration 36.6 months and there were 20 females and 4 males. The six groups were well matched. On these final 24 patients, 1 withdrew due to a severe headache after taking one 400 mg dose of tiaprofenic acid on the first day of the second treatment period. She had previously been very successfully treated with 600 mg daily tiaprofenic acid and had not wished to change her treatment. She had of course been unaware of which treatment she was receiving during the study. A second patient had a rash whilst taking 1.2 g daily tiaprofenic acid and was changed early from this treatment to the next treatment period. This was in fact the 600 mg daily dose and no further rash occurred. Analysis was thus based on 23 completed patients, but the 24th was included where possible.

Patient compliance was good as measured by the number of tablets taken. In fact, out of a possible maximum of 84 tablets the lowest mean fortnightly consumption was 72.6 and the highest 77.5. Serum level estimation of tiaprofenic acid revealed that 5 patients had little or no demonstrable evidence of the drug in their serum. However, separate analysis of these 5 pa-

Table I. Mean visual analogue pain scores at end of each treatment period

	Pain at rest	Pain on movement	Night pain
Placebo	46.8	63.1	42.7
600 mg	33.3	47.5	36.0
n	23	23	23
Wilcoxon matched pairs signed ranks test	p <0.05	p <0.01	NS
Placebo	46.8	63.1	42.7
1.2 g	22.7	38.7	26.0
n	23	23	23
Wilcoxon matched pairs signed ranks test	p <0.001	p <0.001	p <0.01
600 mg	32.0	45.7	34.7
1.2 g	21.9	37.1	25.0
n	24	24	24
Wilcoxon matched pairs signed ranks test	p <0.01	p =0.0503	p =0.0516

tients showed the same results and trends as the rest of the patients studied. One possible explanation is that the sampling occurred too long after the last dose of the drug for serum levels to be detected.

Table I shows the mean visual analogue pain scales. In relief of resting pain tiaprofenic acid was significantly better than placebo on both doses of the drug and the 1.2 g dose was superior to the 600 mg dose. In the relief of pain on movement again both doses were significantly better than placebo and the difference between the two doses was almost significant in favour of the higher dose. However, for night pain only the 1.2 g dose was significantly better than placebo although the pain score was lower on 600 mg than on placebo. Again, the difference between the two doses was almost significant.

Pain scores calculated from the 4 point scale (where 1 = none, 2 = mild, 3 = moderate, 4 = severe) showed the same trend (table II). For resting pain, 1.2 g was significantly better than placebo but 600 mg was not and the difference between the two doses approached significance. Relief of pain on movement showed a similar trend but there was no significant difference between the two doses. Nor was there any significant difference between the two doses for night pain, each approaching significance when compared with placebo.

The mean number of rescue analgesic tablets taken was 19.8 on the 1.2 g dose, 16.5 on the 600 mg dose and 32.8 on placebo. At both doses, when compared with placebo this difference is significant at the 5% level. The mean du-

Table II. Pain scores based on overall assessment at each treatment period

	Pain at rest	Pain on movement	Night pain
Placebo	2.68	3.18	2.73
600 mg	2.41	2.86	2.36
n	22	22	22
Wilcoxon matched pairs signed ranks test	NS	NS	$p = 0.0593$
Placebo	2.63	3.16	2.74
1.2 g	2.00	2.63	2.32
n	19	19	19
Wilcoxon matched pairs signed ranks test	$p < 0.01$	$p < 0.05$	$p = 0.0593$
600 mg	2.33	2.71	2.33
1.2 g	1.96	2.57	2.24
n	21	21	21
Wilcoxon matched pairs signed ranks test	$p < 0.05$	NS	NS

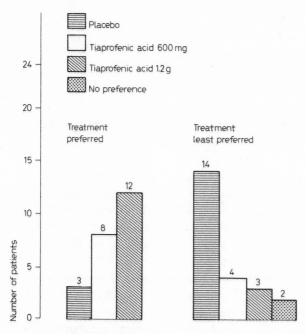

Fig. 1. Patients' preferences.

Table III. Details of side-effects

	Tiaprofenic acid		Placebo
	1.2 g	600 mg	
Gastrointestinal			
Indigestion	2		
Heartburn		1	
Stomach ache/abdominal pain	2		2
Diarrhoea/loose bowels	1		1
Nausea	1		
CNS			
Headache	1	1	1
Sweating		1	1
Giddiness			1
Cutaneous			
Rash on face and swollen neck	1		
Spots on arms and chest			1
Miscellaneous			
Burning sensation in throat	1		
Swollen puffy eyes		1	
Pain under shoulder			1
Chest pain		1	
Total	9	5	8

ration of morning stiffness was 7.6 min prior to treatment, 5.4 min following both placebo and 600 mg and 6.1 min after 1.2 g. Improvement could not be expected with such low initial values.

Patient preferences are shown in figure 1. Most patients preferred treatment with one or other of the two doses of tiaprofenic acid and 1.2 g was preferred most often. The result was significant in favour of the higher dose ($p < 0.05$) when compared with placebo for the most preferred treatment. What patients least preferred shows a mirror of this, placebo being significantly more often the least preferred treatment ($p < 0.05$). Details of side effects are given in table III. These were mostly mild but there was a higher incidence of gastrointestinal intolerance on 1.2 g of tiaprofenic acid. There was no other difference between drug and placebo in terms of side effects. Analysis of the biochemical data showed a trend upwards but remained well within the normal range for both SGOT and γ-GT on 1.2 g only (table IV).

Table IV. Mean SGOT (AST) and γ-GT levels

	n	Mean SGOT, IU/l (normal range: 10–50 IU/l)	n	Mean γ-GT, IU/l (normal range: < 45 IU/l male, < 35 IU/l female)
Baseline	21	20.3	20	23.3
Placebo	21	22.2	19	20.9
600 mg	18	22.6	18	24.2
1.2 g	19	30.7	18	26.6

Discussion

Previous clinical work has shown 600 mg to be an effective and well-tolerated dose of tiaprofenic acid in the treatment of osteoarthritis [3, 4, 6]. This study confirms these findings and shows that a higher dose of 1.2 g daily tiaprofenic acid is more effective than the 600 mg dose. Whether or not the upwards trend in SGOT and γ-GT levels has any clinical significance is hard to assess on the basis of a short-term 2-week crossover study and further chronic data will need to be collected on this. Although upper gastrointestinal complaints were more frequent on the 1.2 g they were mostly mild and in no case was it necessary to discontinue treatment for this reason. Whilst 600 mg is a satisfactory dose for some patients there may be others who will benefit from a higher dose of the drug.

On the basis of this study, and others carried out by the authors, morning stiffness does not appear to be a major problem in osteoarthritis and we would question the value of measuring it. This again raises the discussion about the systemic possibilities of osteoarthritis. The fact that there was little or no demonstrable evidence of the drug in the serum of 5 patients who nevertheless showed the same clinical results highlights the fact that clinical efficacy lasts longer than drug serum levels can be detected and emphasises the difficulty of determining frequency of dosage based on blood levels.

References

1   Berry, H.; Huskisson, E.C.: Treatment of rheumatoid arthritis – use of visual analogue scale. J. clin. Trials *9:* 13–15 (1972).

2   Clemence, F.; Le Martret, O.; Fournex, R.; Plassard, G.; Dagnaux, M.: Recherche de composes anti-inflammatoires et analgesiques dans la serie thiophere. Eur. J. med. Chem. *9:* 390–396 (1974).

3   Thompson, M.; Daymond, T.J.; Essigman, W.K.; Huskisson, E.C.; Wojtulewski, J.A.:
     Short-term efficacy and tolerance of tiaprofenic acid (Surgam) in rheumatoid arthritis and
     osteoarthritis – multi-centre placebo controlled trials. Proc. Monaco Symp. in New Trends
     in Osteoarthritis.
4   Van Eslande, P.: Comparative double-blind study of tiaprofenic acid and indomethacin
     in the treatment of osteoarthritis of the hip. Ars Med., Wien *35:* 1393–1402 (1980).
5   Ward, G.T.; Stead, J.A.; Freeman, M.: A rapid and specific method for the determination
     of tiaprofenic acid in human plasma. J. Liquid Chromatogr. (in press, 1981).
6   Wojtulewski, J.A.; Walter, J.; Thornton, E.J.: Tiaprofenic acid (Surgam) in the treatment
     of osteoarthritis of the knee and hip. Rheumatol. Rehabil. *20:* 177–180 (1981).

H. Berry, MRCP, Department of Rheumatology, King's College Hospital, Denmark Hill,
London SE5 9RS (England)

Rheumatology, vol. 7, pp. 125–135 (Karger, Basel 1982)

Short-Term Efficacy and Tolerance of Tiaprofenic Acid (Surgam) in Rheumatoid Arthritis and Osteoarthritis

Multicentre Placebo-Controlled Trials

M. Thompson[a], T.J. Daymond[b], W.K. Essigman[c], E.C. Huskisson[d], J.A. Wojtulewski[e, 1]

[a] Department of Rheumatology, Royal Victoria Infirmary, Newcastle upon Tyne;
[b] Department of Rheumatology, District General Hospital, Sunderland, Tyne and Wear; [c] Department of Rheumatology, Lister Hospital, Stevenage, Hertfordshire; [d] Department of Rheumatology, St. Bartholomew's Hospital, London; [e] Department of Rheumatology, St. Mary's Hospital, Eastbourne, Sussex, England

Introduction

Tiaprofenic acid [α-(5-benzoyl-2-thienyl)-propionic acid] has been shown in animal studies to be a potent anti-inflammatory and non-narcotic analgesic [2, 3]. Comparative clinical studies have further confirmed that tiaprofenic acid is as effective and at least as well tolerated as phenylbutazone in the treatment of rheumatoid arthritis [1], as ibuprofen in the treatment of rheumatoid arthritis [4], and as indomethacin in the treatment of osteoarthritis [8, 9]. However, it was considered necessary to establish definitive proof of efficacy in these indications by comparing tiaprofenic acid with placebo in stringent double-blind trials. This paper presents the results of two such placebo-controlled trials of tiaprofenic acid conducted to identical therapeutic programmes and methods, one trial in patients suffering from rheumatoid arthritis, the other in patients suffering from osteoarthritis. To the best of our belief this is unique in the investigation of non-steroidal anti-inflammatory drugs.

[1] We are grateful to the Editor of Rheumatology and Rehabilitation for permission to publish this paper.

Design and Measurements

Design

Tiaprofenic acid was compared to placebo in two multicentre crossover trials to an identical design, one in rheumatoid arthritis, the other in osteoarthritis. After a pretrial washout of at least 2 days during which all non-steroidal anti-inflammatory drugs were withdrawn, each patient received 7 days treatment with tiaprofenic acid (200 mg three times a day) and 7 days treatment with placebo in crossover fashion. Free access to escape analgesic tablets (paracetamol 500 mg) was allowed throughout the trial.

Treatments were administered double-blind according to a predetermined randomization schedule which was balanced for each centre. Each investigator was supplied with a sealed envelope for each patient containing the individual treatment order. Envelopes were only to be opened in an emergency. Patients with active peptic ulceration, severe hepatic or renal disease were excluded, as were those receiving anticoagulants, oral hypoglycaemic or immunosuppressive drugs.

Measurements

In both trials the patients were assessed at the end of the pretrial washout and at the end of each treatment period. The efficacy of the treatments was assessed by estimations of pain (10 cm visual analogue scale), consumption of escape analgesic tablets, duration of morning stiffness, articular index – Ritchie et al. [7] in the rheumatoid arthritis trial; Doyle et al. [5] in the osteoarthritis trial –, investigator's overall assessment of response, and patients' preference. In addition the patients completed daily diaries recording pain (10 cm visual analogue scale) and duration of morning stiffness.

Side-effects were elicited by a simple non-leading question, namely: 'Has the treatment during the past week upset you in any way?' 23 routine haematology and serum biochemistry tests were performed in each patient at the end of the washout and at the end of each treatment period. Compliance was estimated from returned tablet counts.

Statistical Analyses

Pain level, consumption of escape analgesic, duration of morning stiffness, and articular index score were analyzed using Student's paired t test. Pain level data were transformed by arc sine transformation prior to analysis. The investigator's overall assessments of response and the patients' preferences were analyzed using the large sample equivalent of the sign test.

Rheumatoid Arthritis Trial

Patients

80 adult patients with active rheumatoid arthritis (ARA criteria) of more than 6 months duration, attending rheumatology outpatient clinics, entered the trial, 20 patients at each of four centres. Patients receiving gold, penicillamine, or corticosteroids were eligible provided that their doses of these drugs had been constant during the 6 months prior to the trial and remained constant throughout the trial.

Of the 80 patients entered, 5 failed to complete, 2 being withdrawn because of side-effects while receiving, placebo, 1 defaulting, 1 being unassessable because of bad compliance, and 1

Table I. Demography of patients in the rheumatoid arthritis trial

	Treatment group	
	tiaprofenic acid/ placebo	placebo/ tiaprofenic acid
Total number of patients	39	36
Sex		
Males	7	4
Females	32	32
Age, years[1]	53.8±12.2	54.4±13.1
Years of rheumatoid arthritis[1]	10.6±10.4	9.1±7.7
ARA classification		
Classical	26	22
Definite	13	14
Rheumatoid factor		
Positive	2	21.
Negative	7	11
Not recorded	5	4
Concomitant rheumatoid arthritis medication		
Gold	0	1
Penicillamine	3	4
Corticosteroid	2	7
Pain level, mm[1]	56.7±19.4	56.2±20.5
Duration of morning stiffness, min[1]	102.8±85.2	106.9±115.5
Ritchie articular index score[1]	18.6±11.7	19.3±8.3

[1] Mean ± SD values.

suffering from a coincident and unrelated illness. The 75 patients who completed the trial were included in the analyses of compliance and efficacy. The demography of these 75 patients is shown in table I. The two treatment order groups were demographically comparable.

Results

Tiaprofenic acid was superior to placebo in all measures, and the differences were statistically highly significant ($p < 0.001$). Results of assessments of pain, escape analgesic consumption, duration of morning stiffness, and articular index recorded at the end of each treatment period are given in table II.

Investigator's overall assessments of responses to both treatments were recorded for 69 patients. The results are given in table III. Overall, tiaprofenic acid was assessed as superior to placebo in 40 patients (58%), equivalent to placebo in 18 patients (26%), and inferior to placebo in 11 patients (16%). This

Table II. Results of post-treatment assessments of pain, escape analgesic consumption, duration of morning stiffness, and articular index in the rheumatoid arthritis trial (mean ± SEM)

	Treatment group	
	tiaprofenic acid	placebo
Pain level, mm	41.4±3.0	51.2±3.0
Significance	$p < 0.001$	
Consumption of escape analgesic	18.0±2.0	23.5±2.0
Significance	$p < 0.001$	
Duration of morning stiffness, min	68.4±8.2	85.1±10.2
Significance	$p < 0.001$	
Ritchie articular index score	14.8±1.2	18.1±1.3
Significance	$p < 0.001$	

Table III. Investigator's overall assessments in the rheumatoid arthritis trial

Response to treatment	Number of patients	
	triaprofenic acid	placebo
Excellent	5	2
Good	29	16
Fair	21	16
Poor	8	17
Very poor	6	18

result was highly statistically significant in favour of tiaprofenic acid ($p < 0.001$).

The patients preference was similar. Of the 74 patients who recorded a response, 45 patients (61%) expressed a preference for tiaprofenic acid, 13 patients (18%) expressed no preference for either treatment, and 16 patients (21%) expressed a preference for placebo. Again, the result was statistically highly significant in favour of tiaprofenic acid ($p < 0.001$).

The results of patients daily assessments of pain (fig. 1) and duration of morning stiffness (fig. 2) reflected the weekly assessments. Compared with placebo tiaprofenic acid reduced values for both parameters on each of the 7 days, significantly so from day 1 in respect of pain and from day 3 in respect of duration of morning stiffness.

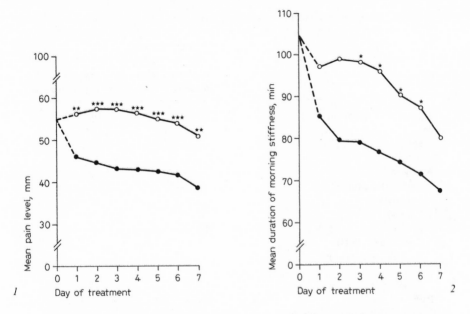

Fig. 1. Pain level (visual analogue scale). ○ = Placebo; ● = tiaprofenic acid. **p < 0.01; ***p < 0.001.

Fig. 2. Duration of morning stiffness. ○ = Placebo; ● tiaprofenic acid. *p < 0.05.

None of the sealed envelopes were opened during the crossover trial. Any patient who took less than 14 of the proposed 21 trial tablets in either week of the trial was excluded from the analyses. Compliance, as estimated from returned tablet counts, was similar for the two treatments. The mean weekly consumption of trial tablets was 20.1 for tiaprofenic acid and 20.2 for placebo.

Osteoarthritis Trial

Patients

60 adult patients with osteoarthritis attending hospital rheumatology out-patient clinics entered the trial, 20 patients at each of three centres. Diagnosis of osteoarthritis was confirmed by radiological features and had been present for at least 6 months.

Of the 60 patients entered only 1 failed to complete the trial. This patient was admitted to hospital for an acute and unrelated illness. The 59 patients who completed the trial were included in the analyses of compliance and efficacy. The demography of these 59 patients is shown in table IV. The two treatment order groups were demographically comparable with the exception that patients in treatment order group 2 (placebo/tiaprofenic acid) had been suffering

Table IV. Demography of patients in the osteoarthritis trial

	Treatment group	
	tiaprofenic acid/ placebo	placebo/ tiaprofenic acid
Total number of patients	30	29
Sex		
Males	9	13
Females	21	16
Age, years[1]	63.1±7.3	62.1±9.5
Years of osteoarthritis[1]	4.3±3.3	7.4±6.0
Joints involved		
Knee(s)	4	4
Hip(s)	11	15
Knee(s) and Hip(s)	2	1
Knee(s) and ankle(s)	2	0
Elbow	0	1
Generalized	11	9
Pain level, mm[1]	50.6±19.8	42.3±22.0
Duration of morning stiffness, min[1]	45.0±67.3	55.8±97.5
Doyle articular index score[1]	11.5±10.1	9.4±9.1

[1] Mean ± SD values.

from osteoarthritis for significantly longer ($p < 0.05$) than patients in treatment order group 1 (tiaprofenic acid/placebo).

Results

The results were similar to those in patients with rheumatoid arthritis. Assessments of pain, escape analgesic consumption, duration of morning stiffness, and articular index recorded at the end of each treatment period are given in table V. Overall tiaprofenic acid was superior to placebo in pain relief and in the number of escape analgesic tablets required, and the differences were statistically highly significant ($p < 0.001$). Tiaprofenic acid was superior to placebo in duration of morning stiffness and articular index and the differences were statistically significant ($p < 0.05$).

Investigator's overall assessments of responses to both treatments were recorded for 56 patients. The results are given in table VI. Overall tiaprofenic acid was assessed as superior to placebo in 40 patients (72%), equivalent to placebo in 12 patients (21%), and inferior to placebo in 4 patients (7%). This result was highly significant in favour of tiaprofenic acid ($p < 0.001$).

Table V. Results of post-treatment assessments of pain, escape analgesic consumption, duration of morning stiffness, and articular index in the osteoarthritis trial (mean ± SEM)

	Treatment group	
	tiaprofenic acid	placebo
Pain level, mm	33.0±3.4	46.4±3.5
Significance	$p < 0.001$	
Consumption of escape analgesic	13.7±2.1	20.1±2.1
Significance	$p < 0.001$	
Duration of morning stiffness, min	30.0±4.6	47.4±8.4
Significance	$p < 0.05$	
Doyle articular index score	9.4±1.6	10.9±1.3
Significance	$p < 0.05$	

Table VI. Investigator's overall assessments in the osteoarthritis trial

Response to treatment	Number of patients	
	tiaprofenic acid	placebo
Excellent	11	1
Good	20	6
Fair	20	17
Poor	3	27
Very poor	2	5

The patients preference was similar. All 59 patients recorded a response. 48 patients (81%) expressed a preference for tiaprofenic acid, 7 patients (12%) expressed no preference for either treatment, and 4 patients (7%) expressed a preference for placebo. Again, the result was statistically highly significant in favour of tiaprofenic acid ($p < 0.001$).

The results of patients daily assessments of pain (fig. 3) and duration of morning stiffnes (fig. 4) reflected the weekly assessments. Tiaprofenic acid reduced values for both parameters on each of the 7 days, significantly so from day 2 onwards.

None of the sealed envelopes was opened during the crossover trial. All patients took at least 14 of the proposed 21 trial tablets in each week of the trial. Compliance, as estimated from returned tablet counts, was similar for the two treatments. The mean weekly consumption of trial tablets was 20.9 for tiaprofenic acid and 20.8 for placebo.

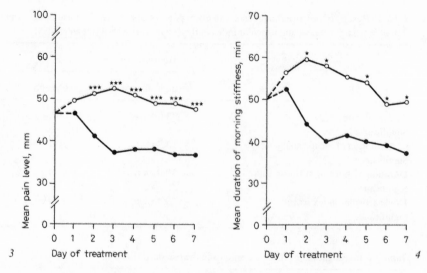

Fig. 3. Pain level (visual analogue scale). O = Placebo; ● = tiaprofenic acid. ***p < 0.001.
Fig. 4. Duration of morning stiffness. O = Placebo; ● = tiaprofenic acid. *p < 0.05.

Table VII. Summary of incidence of side-effects

	Treatment group	
	tiaprofenic acid	placebo
Number of patients assessable	136	138
Number of patients reporting side-effects	31 (23%)	29 (21%)
Number of symptoms reported	36	32
Number of patients withdrawn because of possible side-effects	0	2

Tolerance – Both Trials Combined

Analysis of tolerance was based upon the 140 patients in two trials. Haematological and biochemical tests showed similar results in the tiaprofenic
acid and placebo periods. The incidence and nature of side-effects was similar for the two treatments. Possible side-effects were reported by 23% of patients with tiaprofenic acid and 21% of patients with placebo (table VII).
Symptoms were predominantly mild, and the majority for both treatments
were related to the gastrointestinal system (table VIII). The 2 patients who
were withdrawn because of possible side-effects were both receiving placebo.

Table VIII. Incidence of individual side-effects

Symptoms	Number of reports	
	tiaprofenic acid	placebo
Gastrointestinal		
Nausea	7	5
Dyspepsia	4	6
Abdominal pain	3	3
Heartburn	3	1
Vomiting	1	2[a]
Constipation	1	2
Diarrhoea/loose stools	2	1[a]
Total	21	20
Central nervous system		
Headache	2	4
Drowsiness	3	1
Dizziness	1	1
Depression	0	1
Total	6	7
Miscellaneous		
Sweating	2	1
Rash	1	0
Pruritus	0	1
Blurred vision	1	0
Strange sensation in eyes	1	0
Eyes sensitive to light	0	1
Palpitations	1	1
Tremors	1	1
Vaginal discharge	1	0
Earache	1	0
Total	9	5

[a] 2 patients withdrawn for severe symptoms.

Discussion

These two identical trials have shown that tiaprofenic acid was significantly more effective than placebo and as well tolerated in the treatment of both rheumatoid arthritis and osteoarthritis. They have also shown that tiaprofenic acid had a rapid onset of action, its beneficial effects being evident on the 1st day of treatment in rheumatoid arthritis and on the 2nd day of treatment in osteoarthritis.

Differences between tiaprofenic acid and placebo were similar in the rheumatoid arthirits and osteoarthritis groups. They included significant changes in the duration of morning stiffness, traditionally regarded as a feature of inflammatory arthropathies. This suggests that the drug exerts a useful anti-inflammatory action in both rheumatoid arthritis and osteoarthritis.

The question of whether osteoarthritis is predominately a degenerative or an inflammatory arthropathy continues to be the subject of controversy and debate. However, there now seems little doubt that an inflammatory element exists in the majority of patients suffering from this condition and that non-steroidal anti-inflammatory drugs are the most appropriate treatment [6]. Since many patients respond differently to anti-inflammatory agents, there is a continuing need for effective and well-tolerated alternatives. One such alternative would appear to be tiaprofenic acid.

References

1   Camp, A.V.: Tiaprofenic acid in the treatment of rheumatoid arthritis. Rheumatol. Rehabil. *20:* 181–183 (1981).
2   Clemence, F.; Le Martret, O.; Fournex, R.; Plassard, G.; Dagnaux, M.: Recherche de composes anti-inflammatoires et analgésiques dans la série du tiophene. Eur. J. med. Chem., chim. ther. *9:* 390–396 (1974).
3   Deraedt, R.; Jouquey, S.; Delevallee, F.; Flahaut, M.: Release of prostaglandins E and F in an algogenic reaction and its inhibition. Eur. J. Pharmacol. *61:* 17–24 (1980).
4   Daymond, T.J.; Thompson, M.; Akbar, F.A.; Chestney, V.: A controlled trial of tiaprofenic acid versus ibuprofen in rheumatoid arthritis. Rheumatol. Rehabil. *18:* 257–260 (1979).
5   Doyle, D.V.; Dieppe, P.A.; Scott, J.; Huskisson, E.C.: An articular index for the assessment of osteoarthritis. Ann. rheum. Dis. *40:* 75–78 (1981).
6   Huskisson, E.C.: Routine drug treatment of rheumatoid arthritis and other rheumatic diseases. Clin. rheum. Dis. *5:* 703 (1979).
7   Ritchie, D.M.; Boyle, J.A.; McInnes, J.M.; Jasani, M.K.; Dalakos, T.G.; Grieveson, P.;

Buchanan, W.W.: Clinical studies with an articular index for the assessment of joint tenderness in patients with rheumatoid arthritis. Q.Jl. Med. *37:* 393–406 (1968).

8   Van Eslande, P.: Comparative double-blind study of tiaprofenic acid and indomethacin in the treatment of osteoarthritis of the hip. Ars med. *35:* 1393–1402 (1980).

9   Wojtulewski, J.A.; Walter, J.; Thornton, E.J.: Tiaprofenic acid (Surgam) in the treatment of osteoarthritis of the knee and hip. Rheumatol. Rehabil. *20:* 177–180 (1981).

M. Thompson, MD, Department of Rheumatology, Royal Victoria Infirmary, Queen Victoria Road, Newcastle upon Tyne (England)

Rheumatology, vol. 7, pp. 136–142 (Karger, Basel 1982)

Clinical Trial of Tiaprofenic Acid in Rheumatoid Arthritis with Scintigraphic Study

G. Katona, R. Burgos Vargas, A. Zimbrón

Rheumatology Service, Hospital General de la SSA, Mexico

In testing the anti-inflammatory effect of new drugs, the use of methods which permit the objective measurements as well as the comparison of the inflammatory state before and after the administration of the drug, is of great importance.

Since 1965 [1], radioisotopes with short half-lives have been used because of their capacity to concentrate in inflamed tissue. Technetium pertechnectate (^{99m}Tc) proved to be the most useful and easiest to handle because of its half-life of 6 hours [2, 3, 4, 5, 6]. According to our current knowledge, the greater concentration of radioisotopes in inflamed joints is due, on one hand, to the increased vascularization and on the other, to the enhancement of permeability of the capillary walls of the synovial membrane [9]. The radioisotope reaches the membrane and binds to the inflamed tissue in a greater proportion than it does to non-inflamed tissue [7]. This increase is directly related to the degree of inflammation [10].

Some authors [8] question the usefulness of joint scintigraphy as an objective method in determining the degree of the inflammatory state, and therefore, as a means to measure the anti-inflammatory effect of drugs. The main reason being that the evaluation of the changes observed in the density of the images depends on the observer's subjective impression. By using a densitometer we can sometimes assess more accurately the possible differences in uptake by the inflamed tissues in different areas or on different occasions.

Recently, by using the absorption and distribution curves of the radioisotope as well as the absolute counts of the accumulated radioactivity recorded for 30 min on the different 'areas of interest', we developed an objective and quantitative method for the assessment of joint inflammation [11, 12].

In this study we used joint scintigraphy in a sequential and quantitative way to assess the anti-inflammatory effect of tiaprofenic acid, a new non-stereoidal anti-inflammatory compound, in rheumatoid arthritis patient.

Materials

10 female patients with active Classical Rheumatoid Arthritis according to the ARA criteria [13] with no previous anti-inflammatory therapy were selected for the trial. All of them showed involvement of hands and knees at least with pain, swelling and limited function.

Method

At the time of selection all patients had clinical and laboratory examinations, including the total number of painful and swollen joints as well as duration of morning stiffness. Joint scintigraphy of the hands and knees was performed, and the administration of tiaprofenic acid, 200 mg t.i.d. was started. The overall duration of the study was 4 months.

During the whole trial, patients were examined every 2 weeks clinically as outlined before. Joint scintigraphy was performed at the end of the second and fourth months. The patients were asked during each visit about possible undesirable drug-related effects. Both the investigator's and patient's opinions were recorded.

As already mentioned, before the treatment was started and twice during the study, joint scintigraphy with ^{99m}Tc-pertechnectate was performed. Five mCi of ^{99m}Tc-pertechnectate were administered intravenously and by using a Picker 4c/15 Dynacamera, the uptake and distribution of the radioisotope in 'areas of interest' in the wrist and knee joints were continuously recorded on a videotape for 30 min. Immediately after completion of the study, scans of the involved joints were taken from the videotape. Computerized curves of the radioisotope uptake in the studied joints were also performed. The overall accumulated radioactivity within 30 min in the explored areas and the speed of fixation were considered as quantitative elements.

The total counts were compared before and after the fourth month of treatment and the difference was estimated as a percentage in each joint. In order to estimate the statistical differences related to the clinical results, the Student's t test was used.

Results

Of the 10 selected patients, 7 completed the trial (2 have not finished and 1 defaulted).

From the clinical point of view, most of them showed a marked improvement. The number of painful joints decreased from 21.0 to 2.83 (p<0.001) and the swollen joints from 8.1 to 0.42 (p<0.01) after four months of treat-

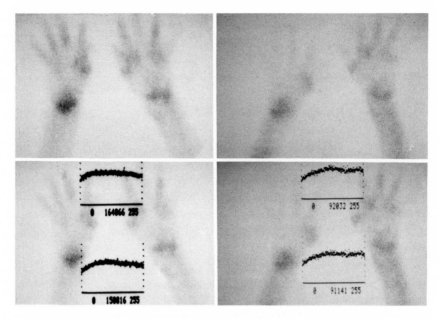

Fig. 1. FOR, 53-year-old female. Dg. active classic rheumatoid arthritis. Hand scintigraphy, concentration curve and total count of radioactivity uptake in the wrist (areas of interest), before (10–10–80) and after (18–12–80) tiaprofenic acid treatment.

ment. The duration of morning stiffness diminished from 37 min to 5 min (p<0.01). Undesirable effects were only reported in 3 cases (one headache, 2 epigastric pains). These effects were only mild and occasional. No changes were reported in the laboratory tests.

The overall assessment reported by the investigator was: 2 very good, 4 good and 1 fair. The patient's own assessment was: three very good, another three good and in one case the patient did not report any improvement. When analyzing the scintigraphies one can observe, in most of them, visible changes in the density of the concentration of the radioisotope in the involved areas, but it is not always related to the total counts. Based on this data in all but one of the recorded joints, a measurable decrease was observed. In some cases the decrease was of 50% or more. To illustrate our findings we selected some of the patients as follows:

Case 2. FOR. A 53-year-old female, with classical rheumatoid arthritis of 2 years duration, showed a good clinical response. In the hand scintigra-

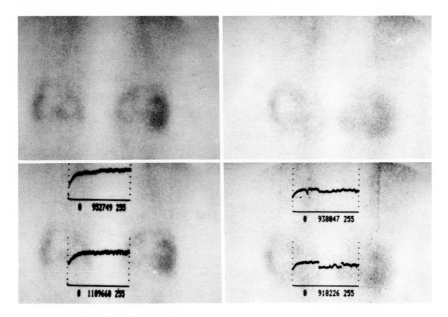

Fig. 2. MLC, 38-year-old female. Dg. active classic rheumatoid arthritis. Knee scintigraphy, concentration curve and total count of radioactivity uptake in the knees (area of interest) before (10–10–80) and after (3–11–81) tiaprofenic acid treatment.

phy a 44% decrease in the total count of radioisotopic uptake was found after 4 months of treatment with tiaprofenic acid (200 mg t.i.d.) (fig. 1).

Case 4. MLC. A 38-year-old female, with classical rheumatoid arthritis of 1 year duration, reported a very good clinical response after 4 months of tiaprofenic acid (200 mg t.i.d.). In the knee scintigraphy a decrease of 17.3% of the total radioactivity was observed (fig. 2).

Case 6. AVM. A 48-year-old female, with classical rheumatoid arthritis of 1 ½ years duration, had a very good clinical response with tiaprofenic acid (200 mg t.i.d.) after 4 months. Scintigraphy of the hands showed a decrease of 18% of the total count (fig. 3).

Case 7. CCG. A 30-year-old female, with classical rheumatoid arthritis of 1 year duration, showed excellent progress with tiaprofenic acid treatment (600 mg/day). In the knee scintigraphy a 37% decrease in the total uptake was observed (fig. 4).

These 4 cases are good examples where clinical observation and changes

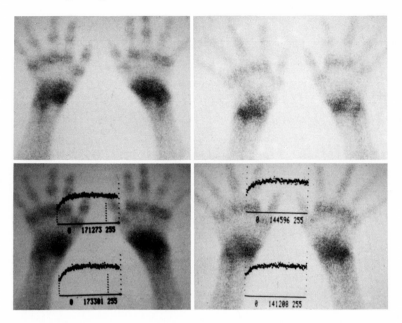

Fig. 3. AVM, 48-year-old female. Dg. active classic rheumatoid arthritis. Hand scintigraphy, concentration curve and total count of radioactivity uptake before (3–16–80) and after (8–10–81) tiaprofenic acid.

in the scintigraphy concurred. In the other three cases the results were more or less similar but the decrease of the uptake in the scintigraphies was found to be more constant and, as mentioned before, only in one joint (case 5) was it absent.

The lack of correlation between the clinical and scintigraphic findings could be explained by several subjective factors which interfere with the clinical assessment as measured by the patient's and investigator's opinions. With quantitative scintigraphy we are looking for a method to detect and measure the anti-inflammatory effect of the drug from a minimum – maybe clinically undetectable – grade to a major decrease of the inflammatory state, in an objective form.

In this study, as measured by the decrease of the accumulated radioactivity in the determined areas of the knees and wrists, tiaprofenic acid had a clear and measurable anti-inflammatory effect. In the clinical measurements, the compound also showed a satisfactory effect and good tolerance.

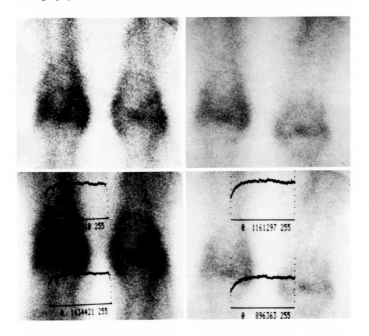

Fig. 4. CCG, 30-year-old female. Dg. active classic rheumatoid arthritis. Knee scintigraphy, concentration curve and total count of radioactivity uptake before (5–30–81) and after (7–30–81) 2 months of treatment with tiaprofenic acid.

References

1   Weiss, T.E.; Maxfield, W.S.; Murison, P.J.; Hidalgo, F.U.: Iodinated human albumin (1–131) localization studies of rheumatoid arthritis joints by scintillation scanning. Arthritis Rheum. *8:* 1976 (1965).

2   Alarcon Segovia, D.; Trujeque, M.; Tovar, E.; Adame, M.A.: Scintillation scanning of joints with technetium 99m. Ann. rheum. Dis. *10:* 262 (1967).

3   Martinez Villaseñor, D.; Bush, P.; Katona, G.: Scintigraphy by means of radioisotopes of short half-life for diagnosing diseases of the joints; in Medical radioisotope scintigraphy, vol. II, p. 295 (International Atomic Energy Agency, Vienna 1965).

4   Roucayrol, J.C.; Delbarre, F.; Ingrand, J.; Aignan, M.: Arthroscintigraphy (scintigraphy of the joints); in Medical radioisotope scintigraphy, vol. II., p. 281 (International Atomic Energy Agency, Vienna 1968).

5   Katona, G.; Martinez, V.D.; Bush, P.: Joint scintigraphy with short-lived radioisotopes and its usefulness compared with X-rays findings in joint diseases. Rev. interam. Rad. *5:* 29 (1970).

6   Maxfield, W.S.; Weiss, T.E.: Technetium [99m] joint images. Radiology *92:* 1961 (1969).

7   McCarty, D.J.; Polcyn, A.E.; Collins, P.A.; Gottschalk, A.: [99m]Technetium scintiphotography in arthritis. I. Technique and interpretation. Arthritis Rheum. *13:* II (1970).

8   McCarty, D.J.; Polcyn, R.E.; Collins, P.A.: [99m] Technetium scintiphotography in arthritis. II. Its non-specificity and clinical and roentgenographic correlations in rheumatoid arthritis. Arthritis Rheum. *13:* 21 (1970).

9   Green, F.A.; Hays, M.J.: The pertechnectate joint scan. Ann. rheum. Dis. *31:* 278 (1972).

10 Katona, G.; Zimbron, A.: The usefullness of radioisotopes in rheumatology. Diagnostic and research experiences – Radioaktive Isotope in Klinik und Forschung, vol. 13, p. 417 (Hegerman, 1978).

11 Whaley, K.; Pack, A.L.; Boyle, J.A.: The articular scan in patients with rheumatoid arthritis: a possible method of quantitating joint inflammation using radio-technetium. Clin. Sci. *35:* 547 (1973).

12 Katona, G.; Burgos Vargas, R.; Zimbron, A.: Sequential quantitative scintigraphy (SQS) using ^{99m}Tc in the follow-up of the anti-inflammatory effect of prioxicam. Wld Conf. Clinical Pharmacology anf Therapeutics, London 1980, abstr. 0835.

13 Ropes, M.W.; Benneth, G.A.; Cobb, S.; Diagnostic criteria for rheumatoid arthritis. Arthritis Rheum. *2:* 16 (1959).

G. Katona, MD, Chief of Rheumatology Service, Hospital General de la SSA, Dr. Balmis No. 148, Mexico, D.F. (Mexico)

Rheumatology, vol. 7, pp. 143–150 (Karger, Basel 1982)

Comparative Study of Tiaprofenic Acid and Diclofenac for the Treatment of Rheumatoid Arthritis

A. Maccagno, P. Santoro

Service of Rheumatology, Hospital Francés, Buenos Aires, Argentina

Introduction

Tiaprofenic acid (Surgam®, Roussel Uclaf) is a nonsteroidal antiinflammatory drug with analgesic properties. Its chemical formula is 5-benzyl-α-methyl-2-thiophene acetic acid (fig. 1). Tiaprofenic acid is a nonspecific antagonist of bradikinine, prostaglandin E_2, serotonin, histamine and acetylcholine. Its antiinflammatory activity is based on the inhibition of prostaglandin synthesis. Previous pharmacological experiments have demonstrated its antiinflammatory efficacy in acute, subacute and chronic conditions. The aim of this test was to determine the clinical efficacy and tolerance of tiaprofenic acid in the treatment of adult rheumatoid arthritis in comparison with diclofenac.

Material and Method

The study was performed on 30 ambulatory patients of both sexes according to a parallel double-blind design, divided into two equal groups receiving treatment during 8 weeks. The patients included in the study suffered from established classic or definite rheumatoid arthritis of the adult as defined by the American Rheumatism Association criteria, in the active phase of the illness. The parameters for defining active illness were the following: (1) number of painful joints on motion: 6 or more; (2) number of swollen joints: 3 or more; (3) duration of morning stiffness: 45 min or more; (4) erythrocyte sedimentation rate (Westergren): 28 mm/h or more.

Patients under treatment with gold salts, penicillamine, immunosuppressive or antimalarial drugs were admitted to the test after 6 months of drug suspension, 1 month after corticosteroids and 1 week after nonsteroidal antiinflammatory treatment. The only other treatment allowed was acetaminophen (500 mg), 1–6 tablets per day, if needed, during the previous week. Strict exclusion criteria were applied.

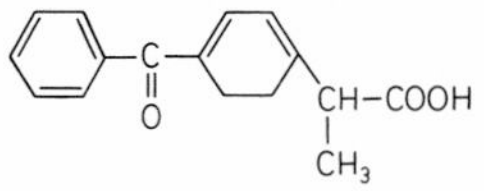

Fig. 1. Chemical formula of tiaprofenic acid.

The drugs were administered according to a previously established random code. Each patient received 8 bottles with an identification with which he entered the study and the week number corresponding to the medication.

The dose was 200 mg, 3 times a day (600 mg/day) for tiaprofenic acid and 50 mg, 3 times a day (150 mg/day) for diclofenac. Both drugs were administered during 8 weeks to each patient.

The parameters for evaluating the activity of each drug were registered on the corresponding check-lists as can be seen from the following scheme:

Visit: 1 2 3 4 5 6 7

Week of treatment: −1 0 1 2 4 6 8

First visit: Selection visit before the treatment. Second visit: Admission visit and start of treatment. Third to sixth visits: Subsequent visits for evaluation. Seventh visit: Final evaluation visit.

The following parameters were evaluated: (1) morning stiffness: duration was expressed in minutes; (2) pain: evaluated according to a 0 to 3 scale (absent, mild, moderate and severe), for each involved joint, at the time of the visit. The articulations examined were: shoulder, elbow, wrist, fingers (distal inter-phalangeal; proximal inter-phalangeal; metacarpo-phalangeal; hip, knee, ankle, tarsal metatarsal, toes (inter-phalangeal proximal; metatarso-phalangeal); (3) swelling: it was determined according to the number of affected joints and a definite intensity scale from 0 to 3 (absent, mild, moderate and severe); (4) functional index: it was evaluated according to the functional capacity for moving and doing usual tasks, using the following scale: 0 = without limitation, 1 = 25% limitation, 2 = 50% limitation, 3 = 75% limitation; (5) grip strength: it was expressed in millimeters of Hg; (6) global evaluation of the clinical sign-symptomatology: according to a previously agreed classification it was rated as marked improvement, improvement and no change; (7) final evaluation: the patient's and investigator's opinions were registered as negative (0), doubtful (1), good (2) or very good (3). These concepts were previously established.

Laboratory examinations (blood and urine) were made before and after treatment. The side effects observed by the physician or spontaneously reported by the patient were also evaluated. The data were statistically evaluated by a Nested Anova analysis and the scores of each visit compared to the score of the first visit by Dunnet's 't' test [1]. Proximal inter-phalangeal joints were considered as one joint, the values being the different inter-phalangeal mean. The same procedure was used for metacarpo-phalangeal and distal inter-phalangeals. This criterion was not employed for the rheumatoid arthritis diagnosis according to ARA.

Results

30 patients entered the study, 15 on tiaprofenic acid and 15 on diclofenac. The treatments distribution was random, double blind. Table I shows

Table I. General characteristics of patients (mean ± SD)

Drug	Patients n	Sex	Age years	Height cm
Tiaprofenic acid	15	7 M 8 F	45.9 ± 11.2	170.7 ± 6.4
Diclofenac	15	4 M 11 F	43.2 ± 12.6	166.3 ± 5.7

Table II. Morning stiffness (number of patients)

Drug	Stiffness min	Visit 1	2	3	4	5	6	7
Tiaprofenic acid	0–10	0	0	0	0	0	0	0
	10–30	1	0	0	1	2	3	4
	30–60	2	3	3	3	4	4	4
	>60	12	12	12	11	9	8	7
Diclofenac	0–10	0	0	0	0	0	0	0
	10–30	0	0	0	0	1	3	3
	30–60	6	5	6	8	8	5	5
	>60	8	9	8	6	5	6	6

Table III. Results of the evaluated parameters

Variable	Drug	Visit 1	2	3	4	5	6	7	DS
Pain[1]	T	8.8	10.4^{**}	9.7	9.4	8.3	7.1^{**}	6.7^{**}	1.2
	D	8.9	9.8	9.4	8.1	7.2^{**}	6.9^{**}	6.4^{**}	
Swelling	T	7.7	9.1^{*}	8.9^{*}	7.9	7.1	6.7	5.7^{**}	1.2
	D	7.9	8.5	8.3	7.6	6.9	6.4^{**}	5.6^{**}	
Functional limitation	T	7.4	8.6	7.7	6.9	6.2	5.6^{**}	4.8^{**}	1.2
	D	6.8	8.1^{*}	7.4	6.6	5.6	5.1^{**}	4.7^{**}	
Grip strength, mm Hg	T	43.21	42.23	43.97	44.47^{*}	47.31^{*}	48.70^{**}	50.95^{**}	3.82
	D	35.42	33.57	34.91	39.11^{*}	41.82^{**}	43.33^{**}	45.43^{**}	

T = Tiaprofenic acid; D = diclofenac; DS = square root of the remainder's mean square of the Nested Anova analysis. $^{*}p < 0.05$; $^{**}p < 0.01$.

[1] Evaluation of parameters = mean of the intensity of the pain concerning all the involved joints at the time of the visit.

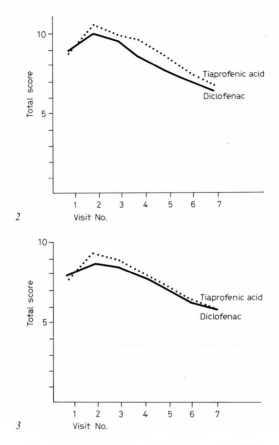

Fig. 2. Pain. DS = 1.2 (for explanation see table III).
Fig. 3. Swelling. DS = 1.2.

the general features of the patients studied. Table II shows the results for morning stiffness. In the group that received tiaprofenic acid, 3 of 5 patients with stiffness on initial evaluation of longer duration than 60 min had, at the final evaluation, a stiffness between 10 and 30 min, and 2 patients were between 30 and 60 min. In the group that received diclofenac, 2 patients with an initial stiffness of longer duration than 60 min and one patient between 30 and 60 min saw their morning stiffness reduced to between 10 and 30 min.

Table III shows the results of pain, swelling, functional limitation and grip strength. The pain diminished significantly ($p < 0.01$) from visit 6 for patients under tiaprofenic acid and from visit 5 for those under diclofenac.

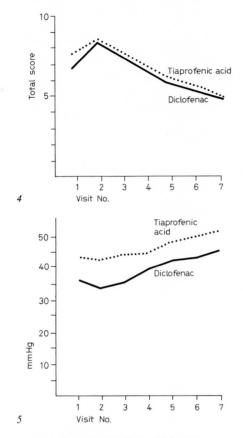

Fig. 4. Functional limitation. DS = 1.2.

Fig. 5. Grip strength.

Figure 2 shows these data graphically. The swelling diminished significantly at visit 7 in the group receiving tiaprofenic acid and at visit 6 in the comparative group (fig. 3). The functional limitation diminished from visit 6 and grip strength increased from visit 5 in both groups (fig. 4 and 5, respectively). No differences were detected between both treatments.

The side effects found in both groups are shown in figure 6. 1 patient of the diclofenac group had to suspend the treatment on account of intolerance (psychophysical asthenia and intense dizziness) on the 5th day. With regard to laboratory analysis (blood and urine) no differences were detected intra and intergroups.

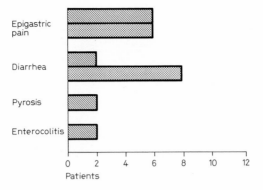

Fig. 6. Side effects. ▨ = Tiaprofenic acid; ▩ = diclofenac.

Table IV. Global evaluation of clinical symptomatology

Group	Marked improvement	Improvement	Total
Tiaprofenic acid	5	7	12
Diclofenac	0	9	9
Total	5	16	21

Difference between groups: $p < 0.05$ (exact probability, Fischer's test).

Table IV represents the global evaluation of the clinical sign symptomatology (last visit), showing the number of cases with marked improvement and improvement in both groups. In the group that received tiaprofenic acid, the number of patients with marked improvement increases with time, this was not the case with the diclofenac group. The final evaluation of the entire treatment period by the physician and the patient (fig. 7) shows a greater number of very good results for tiaprofenic acid as compared with the other treatment and a greater number of doubtful cases under diclofenac. The statistical analysis included 15 patients of the tiaprofenic acid group and 14 receiving diclofenac.

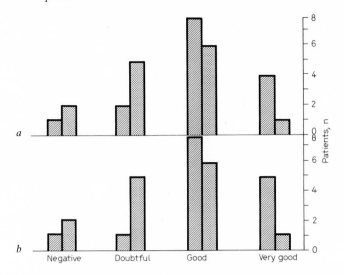

Fig. 7. Final evaluation. *a* = by investigator; *b* = by patient. ▧ = Tiaprofenic acid; ▦ = diclofenac.

Discussion

The statistical evaluation of pain, swelling, functional limitation and grip strength parameters showed a very similar behavior between tiaprofenic acid and diclofenac. The side effects of both drugs were essentially gastro-intestinal in nature. Generally they were transient and clinically negligible. Only 1 case that received diclofenac was dropped from the study because of severe psychophysical asthenia and intense dizziness. The laboratory examinations did not show pathological manifestations due to drug administration in either group. The global evaluation of the clinical symptomatology (last visit) showed that in the group receiving tiaprofenic acid there were 5 cases showing marked improvements against 0 in the diclofenac group; in the 2nd parameter improvement there were 7 cases receiving tiaprofenic acid against 9 for diclofenac. The final evaluation reported by the physician and the patient showed, at a similar level of significance, a greater number of good and very good responses for tiaprofenic acid.

Conclusion

Tiaprofenic acid was shown in this study to be a very efficient safe drug for the treatment of the rheumatoid arthritis.

Summary

The aim of this report is to compare the efficacy of tiaprofenic acid and diclofenac in the treatment of rheumatoid arthritis. Two groups of 15 patients each (random) with classic or definite rheumatoid arthritis (ARA) were studied by the double blind method. Tiaprofenic acid was given in a dose of 200 mg 3 times a day by oral route and diclofenac in a dose of 50 mg 3 times a day orally. This treatment was administered during 8 weeks to each patient. Inclusion and exclusion criteria were those classic for this kind of investigation. Morning stiffness, pain, swelling, functional limitation, grip strength, global symptomatology and final patient's and investigator's appraisal were the parameters evaluated. Laboratory examinations (blood and urine) were made before and after treatment. Side effects detected by the physician or spontaneously reported by the patient were also evaluated. The results obtained were evaluated statistically from a Nested Anova analysis of the data by the Dunnet 't' test.

Conclusions: (1) In this report, tiaprofenic acid (Surgam) has proved to be a useful drug for the treatment of rheumatoid arthritis; (2) the statistical evaluation of the clinical parameters studied – morning stiffness, pain, swelling, functional limitation and grip strength – showed that its effectiveness is similar to diclofenac; (3) the clinical global symptomatology evaluated showed, after 8 weeks of treatment, that in the group receiving tiaprofenic acid, the number of patients with remarkable progress increased significantly. This was not observed in the group receiving diclofenac; (4) the final evaluation of the overall treatment period (based on patient's and investigator's opinion) favoured tiaprofenic acid; (5) tiaprofenic acid was shown to be a well tolerated drug.

Reference

1   Steel, R.G.D.; Torrie, J.H.: Principles and procedures of statistics (McGraw Hill, New York 1960).

A. Maccagno, MD, Julián Alvarez 2749, 3° piso 'A' (1425), Buenos Aires (Argentina)

Rheumatology, vol. 7, pp. 151–158 (Karger, Basel 1982)

Double-Blind Comparative Studies of Tiaprofenic Acid in Degenerative Joint Diseases

J.G. Peyron[1]

Introduction

Tiaprofenic acid (α-[benzoyl-5-thienyl-2]-propionic acid) is a new non-steroidal anti-inflammatory agent. Its activity in patients suffering from degenerative joint disease has been evaluated in a series of multi-center, double-blind, parallel studies. It was first compared with placebo and then with other standard anti-inflammatory drugs, namely acetylsalicylic acid (ASA) ibuprofen and indomethacin. Of the patients who entered these studies, 244 received tiaprofenic acid, 73 placebo, 68 ASA, 63 ibuprofen and 82 indomethacin.

The majority of patients suffered from osteoarthritis (OA) of the hip, the knee, or the cervical or lumbar spine. Comparability of the groups in each study was confirmed. The treatment period was 7 days. Pain and joint mobility were assessed before and after treatment. Pain was reported in four grades in the trial against placebo, ASA and ibuprofen (0 = absent; 1 = mild; 2 = moderate; 3 = severe) and in six grades in the study comparing tiaprofenic acid with indomethacin (0 = absent; 1 = very mild; 2 = mild, 3 = moderate; 4 = severe; 5 = very severe). Joint mobility was also reported in four grades in the first three trials, and in five grades in the indomethacin study. Global results, taking into account effects on pain and mobility, were graded by the physician as very good, good, fair and insufficient or nil. The patients were adult outpatients seen in nine rheumatology clinics throughout the country.

[1] Drs. *Attali, Benichou, Bloch, Michel, Boulet-Gercourt, Camus, Chatelin, Chouraki, Dechelotte, Kaplan, Leca, Mesmin, Paraf, Pouletty, Sejournet, Six, Souplet* have participated in the different studies.

Table I. Tiaprofenic acid vs. placebo: comparability of the groups

	Tiaprofenic acid	Placebo
Number of patients	73	72
Mean age, years	59.9	60.2
Sex ratio F/M + F, %	76	73
Conditions treated		
Lumbar spine syndrome	31	33
Cervical spine syndrome	10	6
Knee OA	13	15
Hip OA	7	6
Painful shoulder	6	6
Miscellaneous	6	6
Pain before treatment		
Severe	18	15
Moderate	53	52
Mild	2	5

Table II. Tiaprofenic acid vs. placebo: clinical results

	Tiaprofenic acid	Placebo
Very good	18	6
Good	21	15
Fair	12	8
Insufficient or nil	22	43
Total	73	72

Pregnant women, patients with a history of peptic ulcer, renal or liver disease, of allergy to ASA or other non-steroidal anti-inflammatory agents were excluded. No other antirheumatic or analgesic agent was given during the 7-day trial period.

Methods

Tiaprofenic Acid vs. Placebo

600 mg/day of tiaprofenic acid was compared to a placebo. Both were given three times a day. 145 patients completed the trial: 73 received tiaprofenic acid and 72 placebo. The groups were evenly matched (table I).

The results are reported in table II: globally, on tiaprofenic acid 52 cases were improved and 22 were not while on placebo 29 patients improved and 43 did not. The effectiveness of the

Table III. Tiaprofenic acid vs. placebo: analysis of variance of pain improvement and of joint mobility improvement

Sources of variance	SC	ddl	V	F	P
Pain improvement					
Treatments	12.80	1	12.80	14.14	0.001
Observers	6.85	7	0.98	1.08	n.s.
Interaction	4.47	7	0.64	0.71	–
Residual	118.57	131	0.91	–	–
Total	142.69	146	–	–	–
Joint mobility improvement					
Treatments	3.63	3	3.63	8.11	0.001
Observers	3.80	7	0.54	1.21	n.s.
Interaction	3.11	7	0.44	0.99	–
Residual	54.58	122	0.45	–	–
Total	65.12	137	–	–	–

Table IV. Tiaprofenic acid vs. placebo: side effects

	Tiaprofenic acid	Placebo
Heartburn, epigastric pain	11	7
Nausea	3	0
Abdominal pain	0	2
Diarrhea	1	0
Pruritic rash	1	0
Malaise, undefined	2	4

The treatment was stopped for gastric symptoms in 4 patients on tiaprofenic acid and 2 patients on placebo.

active treatment is clearly demonstrated. An analysis of variance was carried out on pain improvements and on mobility (table III) which showed a significant improvement in favor of active treatment. Tolerance is reported in table IV. Gastrointestinal tract symptoms occurred in 15 patients on tiaprofenic acid and 9 on placebo. Treatment was stopped, for gastric symptoms, in 4 patients on tiaprofenic acid and 2 on placebo.

Tiaprofenic Acid vs. ASA and Ibuprofen
    The design of the study, the period of treatment (7 days) and the criteria for assessment were the same as in the study against placebo. The daily doses compared were: tiaprofenic acid 600 mg, ASA 2,000 mg, ibuprofen 1,200 mg. 87 patients took tiaprofenic acid, 68 ASA, and 63 ibuprofen. Comparability of the groups is shown in table V.

Table V. Tiaprofenic acid vs. ASA and ibuprofen: comparability of the groups

	Tiaprofenic acid	ASA	Ibuprofen
Number of patients	87	68	63
Mean age, years	57	59	58
Sex ratio F/F + M, %	68.5	73.5	62
Conditions treated			
Cervical spine syndrome	7	4	9
Lumbar spine syndrome	24	16	15
Painful shoulder	12	7	9
Knee OA	11	7	9
Hip OA	10	12	6
Miscellaneous	14	9	8
Pain before treatment			
Severe	24	17	17
Moderate	63	51	46
Mild	0	0	0

Table VI. Tiaprofenic acid vs. and ibuprofen: clinical results

	Tiaprofenic acid	ASA	Ibuprofen
Very good	12 } 43.9%	7 } 42.6%	7 } 39.6%
Good	24	22	18
Fair	15	10	14
Insufficient or nil	36	29	24
Total	87	68	63

The results are reported in table VI. Tiaprofenic acid relieved to some extent 56.8% of patients, 43.9% very well or well, ASA 57.3 and 42.6% and ibuprofen 61.9 and 39.6%, respectively. No significant difference was demonstrated between the three groups. The degree of improvement in the three groups was studied separately for pain and for joint mobility (fig. 1). No significant difference was demonstrated, but there was a somewhat smaller improvement in mobility with ibuprofen. In this study the analysis of variance showed a slight inter-observer effect possibly due to the necessity of comparing the results of three products from nine different centers. Tolerance results are shown in table VII, and summarized for gastrointestinal tract symptoms in table VIII. The differences between the groups are not significant.

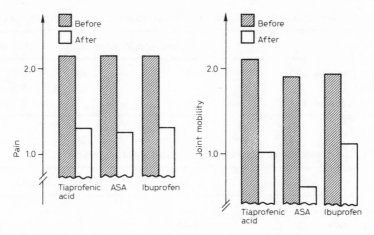

Fig. 1. Mean scores for pain and joint mobility before and after treatment with tiaprofenic acid, aspirin and ibuprofen.

Table VII. Tiaprofenic acid vs. ASA and ibuprofen: side effects

	Tiaprofenic acid		ASA		Ibuprofen	
	treatment maintained	treatment stopped	treatment maintained	treatment stopped	treatment maintained	treatment stopped
Heartburn and gastric pain	6	4	9	2	4	2
Nausea		2	1	2	1	
Abdominal pain	1		1		1	
Rash					1	
Miscellaneous, relation doubtful						
Tinnitus	1					
Excess perspiration					1	
Asthenia	1					
Thoracic pain	1					

Tiaprofenic Acid vs. Indomethacin

Once again the study design and the treatment period were the same. As already mentioned, pain was assessed in six grades and joint mobility in five grades. Only three types of condition were admitted to the trial: OA of the hip knee and cervical spine. The doses compared were 600 mg of tiaprofenic acid and 100 mg of indomethacin. Comparability of the groups is shown in table IX and they appear evenly matched except that the number of female patients is slightly higher in the indomethacin group.

Table VIII. Tiaprofenic acid vs. ASA and ibuprofen: prevalence of gastrointestinal side effects

	Tiaprofenic acid	ASA	Ibuprofen
Number of patients	87	68	63
Side effects	13	15	8
Of which treatment stopped	6	4	2

Table IX. Tiaprofenic acid vs. indomethacin: comparability of the groups

	Tiaprofenic acid	Indomethacin
Number of patients	86	82
Mean age, years	63.6	62.6
Sex ratio F/M + F, %	61.6	70.0
Conditions treated		
Hip OA	28	32
Knee OA	30	25
Cervical spine OA	28	25
Pain level before treatment		
Grade 5	13	15
Grade 4	50	41
Grade 3	23	26

Table X. Tiaprofenic acid vs. indomethacin: clinical results

	Tiaprofenic acid	Indomethacin
Very good	22 } 54.3%	23 } 57.3%
Good	24	24
Fair	17	13
Insufficient or nil	23	22

Results are summarized in table X. In summary, tiaprofenic acid relieved 73% of the patients, 53.4% of whom had good or very good results, the corresponding figures for indomethacin being 73 and 57.4%. The effect on the mean level of pain and joint mobility for each product is represented in figure 2. It is obvious that no difference appears between the drugs. Side effects are shown in table XI. It can be seen that drowsiness and headache, well-known side effects of indomethacin, have not occurred with tiaprofenic acid. The summary of digestive tract side effects appears in table XII and shows only a slight difference between the two agents.

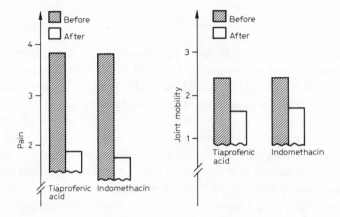

Fig. 2. Mean scores for pain and joint mobility before and after treatment with tiaprofenic acid and indomethacin.

Table XI. Tiaprofenic acid vs. indomethacin: tolerance

	Tiaprofenic acid		Indomethacin	
	treatment maintained	treatment stopped	treatment maintained	treatment stopped
Heartburn and gastric pain	11	2	7	1
Nausea, vomiting	3	2	1	3
Abdominal pain	1		1	
Diarrhea	2		3	
Dizziness	1		2	
Sleepiness			2	
Headache			1	

Table XII. Tiaprofenic acid vs. indomethacin: summary of gastrointestinal tract side effects

	Tiaprofenic acid	Indomethacin
Number of patients	86	82
Side effects	21	16
Of which treatment stopped	4	4

Conclusion

Tiaprofenic acid, 600 mg/day has been compared in five groups of double-blind multi-center studies over 7 days, first with a placebo, and subsequently with ASA (200 mg/day), ibuprofen (1,200 mg/day), and indomethacin (100 mg/day). The condition treated was degenerative joint disease in out-patients. The criteria evaluated were pain level and joint mobility. Comparability of the groups was confirmed.

The comparison with placebo revealed unequivocal therapeutic effectiveness with tiaprofenic acid ($p < 0.01$). No significant differences appeared, under the conditions of the studies between tiaprofenic and the active drugs with which it was compared. During these relatively short treatment periods the side effects of tiaprofenic acid were not noticeably different from those of the comparative agents.

J.G. Peyron, MD, 1, rue Eugène Manuel, F-75016 Paris (France)

Rheumatology, vol. 7, pp. 159–163 (Karger, Basel 1982)

A Short-Term Double-Blind Trial of Tiaprofenic Acid and Naproxen in Osteoarthritis of the Hip

E. Rinaldi, G. Tella

Orthopaedic Department, University of Parma, Parma, Italy

Introduction

Tiaprofenic acid is a non-steroidal, proprionic acid derivative α-(5-benzoyl-2-thienyl)-propionic acid, which has been shown to possess considerable anti-inflammatory and analgesic properties in animals.

These properties have been confirmed in clinical studies in arthritic patients which have shown that tiaprofenic acid has therapeutic effects similar to, or in some cases greater than other anti-inflammatory drugs previously employed, such as acetylsalicylic acid, sulindac, ibuprofen and indomethacin. The drug has been reported to cause no significant changes in body biochemistry nor to cause significant side-effects.

The aim of the study was to evaluate and compare the clinical effects of tiaprofenic acid and naproxen in patients with osteoarthritis of the hip.

Methods

Forty hospitalised patients (33 females and 7 males), aged between 33 and 79 years suffering from unilateral or bilateral hip joint arthrosis where studied. The duration of the disease ranged from 4 months to 30 years. All patients had to satisfy at least three criteria of physical impairment.

Patients with X-ray evidence of third or fourth degree joint lesions (Steinbrocker classification), those with other significant pathology and patients in early pregnancy were exluded from the study as were those receiving steroid or other antipyretic drugs or physiotherapy.

Experimental Design

Each patient taking part in the study received one of the drug treatments and the study was double-blind.

As the shape of the tablets of the preparations to be compared and the administration schedules differed, the double dummy technique was adopted to maintain blindness. All active tablets were given with a placebo identical to the shape and size of the alternative active preparation.

Patients were assigned to treatment according to a randomised table and drug administration was as shown below.

	Morning	Mid-Day	Evening
Tiaprofenic acid (T)	200 mg T	200 mg T	200 mg T
200 mg t. d. s.	+ placebo N	+ placebo N	+ placebo N
Naproxen (N)	250 mg N	placebo N	250 mg N
250 mg bd	+ placebo T	+ placebo T	+ placebo T

Drug treatment was administered for 16 days.

Evaluation of Activity

The following parameters were assessed on days 0, 8 and 16.

1. *Pain.* Spontaneous diurnal pain, spontaneous nocturnal pain, pain on walking, pain after muscular work, and pain on passive movement were each assessed on a 5 point scale of severity.

2. *Mobility.* General mobility was similarly assessed on a 5 point scale.

3. *Walking Time.* Time spent to cover 15 m was recorded in seconds.

4. *Joint Swelling.* The maximal intermalleolar and intercondylar distances were measured in cm.

5. *Morning Stiffness.* The duration of morning stiffness was recorded in minutes.

Evaluation of Tolerability

Possible adverse drug reactions to tiaprofenic acid or naproxen were looked for and recorded during the course of the study.

Statistical Analysis

The following tests were used: Friedman: comparison between the semiquantitative + parameters recorded at each time of observation in each group; the U test of Mann-Whitney: comparison between substances of semiquantitative + parameters recorded at each experimental time; the Skory χ^2 test: comparison between substances of qualitative ++ parameters; Student's test: comparison of quantitative +++ parameters recorded before and after treatment; Variance analysis: comparison of differences of quantitative +++ parameters recorded before and after treatment (+ = different types of pain, total pain index, articular mobility, morning stiffness; ++ = efficacy on pain and on function; +++ = laboratory index).

Table I. Different types of pain considered; significance of time comparison in Friedman test

	Tiaprofenic acid p	Naproxen p
Spontaneous diurnal pain		
Right	< 0.01	< 0.01
Left	< 0.01	< 0.05
Spontaneous nocturnal pain		
Right	< 0.01	< 0.05
Left	< 0.01	< 0.05
Walking pain		
Right	< 0.01	< 0.01
Left	< 0.01	< 0.05
Pain after muscle work		
Right	< 0.01	< 0.01
Left	< 0.01	< 0.05
Passive mobilization pain		
Right	< 0.01	< 0.01
Left	< 0.01	< 0.05

Results

Pain

Pain scores in the five aspects of pain which were monitored were analysed both separately and collectively. In each case tiaprofenic acid gave
greater reduction in pain than naproxen.

Statistical analysis showed that both substances significantly decreased
joint pain. When considering each type of pain separately the Friedman test
shows highly significant relief in the group administered tiaprofenic acid
($p < 0.01$) while in the group receiving naproxen improvement was mostly
significant at the level of $p < 0.05$ (table I).

Considering the cumulative pain index (table II) the differences in general pain index were highly significant for both substances but there was a
lack of significance in the comparison between treatments (U Test Mann-
Whitney).

These results show that the analgesic effect of the two treatments was
very similar but somewhat more evident in the group receiving tiaprofenic
acid.

Table II. Pain general index

Basal		8 days		16 days		Friedman test	
tiaprofenic acid (n = 20)	naproxen (n = 20)	tiaprofenic acid	naproxen	tiaprofenic acid	naproxen	tiaprofenic acid	naproxen
22.75	23.85	17.65	19.20	14.35	16.65	$\chi^2 = 29.2^{**}$	$\chi^2 = 27.3^{**}$
NS	NS	NS	NS	NS	NS	(2 d.f.)	(2 d.f.)

NS = Not significant; $^* = p < 0.05$; $^{**} = p < 0.01$.

Table III. Joint motility

Basal		8 days		16 days		Friedman test	
tiaprofenic acid	naproxen	tiaprofenic acid	naproxen	tiaprofenic acid	naproxen	tiaprofenic acid	naproxen
Right							
2.83	2.74	2.22	2.32	1.78	1.89	$\chi^2 = 15.53^{**}$	$\chi^2 = 12.74^{**}$
(n = 18)	(n = 19)					(2 d.f.)	(2 d.f.)
NS	NS	NS	NS	NS	NS		
Left							
2.33	2.47	1.89	2.24	1.39	1.88	$\chi^2 = 12.86^{**}$	$\chi^2 = 5.85$
(n = 18)	(n = 17)					(2 d.f.)	(2 d.f.) NS
NS	NS	NS	NS	NS	NS		

NS = Not significant; $^* = p < 0.05$; $^{**} = p < 0.01$.

Joint Mobility

Joint mobility was improved after the use of both substances, in the case of tiaprofenic acid significantly on both sides of the body and in the case of naproxen on the left side of the body (table III). There was no significant differences between treatment groups at the 8 and 16 day assessments.

Maximal Intermalleolar Distance, Maximal Intercondylar Distance and Time to Cover 15 m.

No significant difference was found between treatments for any of these parameters.

Morning Stiffness

A significant decrease in the duration of morning stiffness was observed both after tiaprofenic acid ($p < 0.01$) and naproxen ($p < 0.05$). There was no difference between the two treatment groups.

Tolerability

Tiaprofenic acid was very well tolerated there being no gastric, enteric or dermatological side-effects recorded. It should be noted however, that patients with overt gastric disease were excluded from the study.

After naproxen one patient had acute hypertension and another complained of nausea.

Neither treatment affected the haematological parameters which were monitored.

Discussion

Our comparative study between tiaprofenic acid and naproxen has shown tiaprofenic acid to be a very effective analgesic and anti-inflammatory drug as judged by its effects on pain relief and joint mobility in osteoarthritis of the hip. The effects of tiaprofenic acid were indistinguishable from those of naproxen.

Tiaprofenic acid has shown good general and biological tolerance without causing side-effects of any importance.

E. Rinaldi, MD, Orthopaedic Department, University of Parma, via Gramsci 14, I-43100 Parma (Italy)

Rheumatology, vol. 7, pp. 164–172 (Karger, Basel 1982)

Multi-Center Double-Blind Controlled Study of Tiaprofenic Acid versus Indomethacin in the Treatment of Osteoarthritis of the Knee

Takamasa Kageyama

Department of Orthopedic Surgery, Rheumatism and Allergy Center, Sagamihara National Hospital, Sagamihara, Kanagawa, Japan

Introduction

Tiaprofenic acid is a new nonsteroidal anti-inflammatory agent that has been shown to have potent analgesic and anti-inflammatory activities in classic animal models [1]. It has also been demonstrated to be less likely to cause gastrointestinal irritation than indomethacin and other widely used anti-inflammatory agents [1, 2]. Clinical studies have already established the therapeutic efficacy of tiaprofenic acid in treating patients with low back pain [3], neck-shoulder-arm syndrome [4], postoperative pain [5] and post-traumatic pain [6, 7]. In these studies, patient tolerance has been shown to be encouragingly high.

In the present report, in order to evaluate the therapeutic effectiveness, safety and usefulness of tiaprofenic acid in the treatment of osteoarthritis of the knee, we conducted a multi-center double-blind controlled study in 19 institutions using indomethacin as an active control drug based on the double dummy method.

Patients and Method

All the clinics participating in the study used the same protocol and the same case report forms so that as reliable an assessment as possible on treatment response could be achieved with a homogeneous and carefully selected group of patients. Patients with osteoarthritis of the knee were randomly assigned to one of two treatment groups: tiaprofenic acid (TA) 600 mg daily – TA group, and indomethacin (IM) 75 mg daily – IM group, as shown in figure 1. For 1 week prior to the start of the treatment with the test drug, all patients were withdrawn from any preceding drug regimen, and for the following 4 weeks they were administered TA or IM orally in three

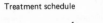

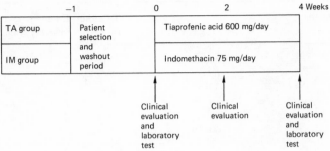

Fig. 1. Multi-center double-blind controlled study of tiaprofenic acid vs. indomethacin in the treatment of osteoarthritis of the knee.

Table I. Examination and evaluation measures

Subjective and objective evaluation
a Pain at rest
b Tenderness
c Pain on passive movement
d Joint swelling
e Difficulty in specific daily activities
   Walking, climbing and getting down stairs, squatting, etc.
f Limitation in flexion and extension of the knee on passive movement
   Rating scale: 0 = none; 1 = slight; 2 = moderate; 3 = marked

Global improvement rating
a Investigator's assessment of overall treatment response in relation to baseline
   Rating scale: 1 = marked improvement; 2 = moderate improvement; 3 = slight improvement; 4 = unchanged; 5 = worse
b Patient's opinion as to overall response to treatment compared with his baseline
   Rating scale: 1 = much better; 2 = better; 3 = slightly better; 4 = unchanged; 5 = worse

Overall usefulness
Investigator's evaluation of overall usefulness based upon a combination of efficacy and safety of the trial drug
   Rating scale: 1 = very useful; 2 = useful; 3 = slightly useful; 4 = usefulness not clear; 5 = undesirable

divided doses after each meal. Osteoarthritis of the knee was selected as the target disease of the study because it is one of the most common forms of osteoarthritis and also because the knee joint, being located near the body surface, permits close observation of the therapeutic response in symptomatology. Diagnostic criteria for patients selection included distinct pain and other inflammatory signs, together with positive X-ray findings. The choice of dosage regimen was based on preliminary open studies which established that 600 mg daily of TA given in three

Table II. Background of patients

Background factor		TA group (n = 91)	IM group (n = 79)	Statistical analysis
Sex	male	22	23	NS[1]
	female	69	56	
Age, years	30–39	2	1	NS[2]
	40–49	10	13	
	50–59	25	21	
	60–69	27	22	
	70–	27	22	
Body weight, kg	–39	0	2	NS[2]
	40–49	15	14	
	50–59	46	37	
	60–69	21	20	
	70–	3	3	
	unknown	6	3	
Duration of disease	–1 weeks	6	4	NS[2]
	–1 month	21	24	
	–3 months	25	21	
	–6 months	14	14	
	–1 year	4	6	
	–3 years	16	9	
	over 3 years	5	1	
Complication[3]	present	15	17	NS[1]
	absent	76	62	
Overall degree of disease activity at week 0	mild	13	11	NS[2]
	moderate	68	58	
	severe	10	10	

divided doses after each meal was the most appropriate dosage [8]. IM is most commonly used in Japan in a dosage of 25 mg given three times daily and this was therefore chosen as the standard comparative agent. No other analgesic or anti-inflammatory drugs were permitted during the course of the study.

Clinical improvement was evaluated based on the following parameters: pain at rest, pain on passive movement, tenderness, joint swelling, interference with daily activities and limitation in flexion and extension of the knee on passive movement (table I). The global improvement rating as measured by the investigator's assessment and the patients' opinion of overall treatment response in relation to the baseline were recorded. Tolerance to therapy was evaluated by questioning the patient and by laboratory studies. At the end of the trial overall usefulness, based upon a combination of efficacy and safety, was also evaluated in each case. A total of 170 patients were considered suitable for evaluation at the end of the study, 91 in the TA group and 79 in the IM group.

Table II. (continued)

Background factor		TA group (n = 91)	IM group (n = 79)	Statistical analysis
Severity of each symptom at week 0[4]				
Pain at rest	0	20	14	NS[2]
	1	23	22	
	2	45	36	
	3	3	7	
Tenderness	0	6	8	NS[2]
	1	39	29	
	2	40	35	
	3	6	7	
Pain on passive movement	0	13	13	NS[2]
	1	32	27	
	2	41	35	
	3	5	4	
Joint swelling	0	20	16	NS[2]
	1	45	41	
	2	25	19	
	3	1	3	
Difficulty in daily activities				
Walking	0	17	15	NS[2]
	1	38	33	
	2	31	28	
	3	5	3	
Climbing and getting down stairs	0	1	0	NS[2]
	1	20	20	
	2	57	51	
	3	13	8	
Squatting	0	1	1	NS[2]
	1	22	15	
	2	50	54	
	3	18	9	
Limitation in motion on passive movement	0	25	31	NS[2]
	1	34	26	
	2	32	19	
	3	0	3	

[1] Chi square test.
[2] Wilcoxon's rank sum test.
[3] Not serious; hypertension, orthopedic (osteoarthrosis of the spine et al.) and others.
[4] 0 = none; 1 = slight; 2 = moderate; 3 = marked.

Table III. Degree of improvement in each symptom at 4 weeks

Symptom[1]	Drug group	Improvement, %			Un-chang-ed, %	Worse %	Total number of pa-tients	Improve-ment rate, % ≥ 2	Statistical analysis	
		marked	moder-ate	slight					Wilcoxon's rank sum test	χ^2 test (≥ 2)
		1	2	3	4	5				
Pain at rest	TA	13	36	35	16	0	71	49	NS	$\chi_0^2 = 4.097$
	IM	9	22	55	14	0	65	31		$p < 0.05$
Tender-ness	TA	6	29	39	25	1	85	35	$Z_0 = 2.337$	$\chi_0^2 = 6.840$
	IM	7	9	46	38	0	71	16	$p < 0.05$	$p < 0.01$
Pain on passive movement	TA	12	19	46	23	0	78	31	$Z_0 = 1.771$	$\chi_0^2 = 3.136$
	IM	6	11	53	30	0	66	17	$p < 0.10$	$p < 0.10$
Joint swelling	TA	4	11	56	27	2	71	15	NS	NS
	IM	5	14	49	32	0	63	19		
Difficulty in daily activities										
Walking	TA	9	18	46	27	0	74	27	NS	NS
	IM	9	16	39	36	0	64	25		
Climbing and getting down stairs	TA	11	30	36	22	1	91	41	$Z_0 = 2.808$	$\chi_0^2 = 6.292$
	IM	10	12	37	40	1	79	22	$p < 0.01$	$p < 0.05$
Squatting	TA	13	25	40	21	1	90	38	$Z_0 = 2.494$	$\chi_0^2 = 8.224$
	IM	9	8	51	32	0	78	17	$p < 0.05$	$p < 0.01$
Limitation of passive movement	TA	5	15	39	41	0	66	20	NS	NS
	IM	0	13	35	52	0	48	13		

[1] Patients who had no symptoms from the beginning to the end of the study are excluded.

Results

An analysis of baseline characteristics, including the severity of each symptom assessed (table II), revealed no significant differences between the two groups. Therefore, it was considered that the two groups were sufficiently homogeneous to ensure a valid comparison of their therapeutic results. The degree of improvement in each individual symptom compared with the baseline was evaluated after 2 and 4 weeks of treatment, and both drug groups showed definite improvement in symptomatology. As shown in table III, the improvement rating after 4 weeks for pain at rest, tenderness and difficulty

Table IV. Final global improvement rating

Drug group	Improvement			Un-chang-ed	Worse	Total number of patients	Improve-ment rate, % ≥ 2	Statistical analysis
	marked	mod-erate	slight					
	1	2	3	4	5			
TA	16 (17)	38 (42)	25 (28)	11 (12)	1 (1)	91	59	Wilcoxon's rank sum test
		(59)	(87)					$Z_0 = 2.970$
								$p < 0.01$
IM	8 (10)	15 (19)	46 (58)	10 (13)	0	79	29	χ^2 test (≥ 2)
		(29)	(87)					$\chi_0^2 = 14.397$
								$p < 0.01$

Figures in parentheses show percent.

Table V. Patients with adverse reactions

	TA group	IM group	Statistical analysis (χ^2 test)
Number of patients evaluated	113	110	
Number of patients with adverse reactions	13 (11.5)	30 (27)	$\chi_0^2 = 7.920$ $p < 0.01$
Number of patients discontinued because of adverse reactions	6 (5)	11 (10)	NS
Severity of adverse reaction			
Mild	8	18	NS
Moderate	3	9	
Severe	2	3	
Gastrointestinal	10 (9)	24 (22)	NS
Stomach pain	2	9	
Nausea/vomiting	4	4	
Others	4	11	
Edema	4 (3.5)	6 (5.5)	
Central nervous system (drowsiness)	3 (3)	3 (3)	
Skin (rash/itching)	0	3 (3)	
Others	1	2	

Figures in parentheses show percent.

Table VI. Overall usefulness rating

Drug group	Very useful	Useful	Slightly useful	Usefulness not clear	Undesirable	Total number of patients	Usefulness rate, %	Statistical analysis
	1	2	3	4	5		$\geqslant 2$	
TA	18	46	10	15	2	91	70	Wilcoxon's rank
	(20)	(50)	(11)	(17)	(2)			sum test
			(70)	(81)				$Z_0 = 3.111$
								$p < 0.01$
								χ^2 test $(\geqslant 2)$
IM	6	27	31	13	2	79	42	$\chi_0^2 = 12.934$
	(8)	(34)	(39)	(16)	(3)			$p < 0.01$
			(42)	(81)				

Figures in parentheses show percent.

in climbing, getting down stairs and in squatting favored the TA group, with statistically significant between-group differences. As can be seen in table IV, the results of the investigator's final global improvement rating of the TA group showed 17% of the patients with marked improvement and 59% with marked to moderate improvement. By comparison, these figures were 10 and 29% in the IM group, respectively. These results show a statistically significant superiority of TA 600 mg over IM 75 mg. TA was also significantly superior to IM in the patients' opinion concerning overall response to treatment. The degree of improvement as measured by the investigator's and the patients' evaluation of overall treatment response tended to progress over time so that on average, maximal improvement occurred at the end of the study in both drug groups.

Side effects, as indicated in table V, developed in 11.5% of the TA-treated patients and 27% of the IM group. The side effect related discontinuation rate was 5% for the TA group and 10% for the IM group. The occurrence of side effects was thus significantly less frequent in the TA group than in the IM group. Gastrointestinal side effects were most commonly encountered in both drug groups. None of the side effects were of a serious nature and there were no significant differences between the two groups in type or degree of severity. When a comparison was made between values of laboratory examinations performed at the beginning and the end of study, there were no changes of statistical or clinical significance, although a slight elevation of SGPT was observed in 1 patient of each drug group.

With regard to overall usefulness, TA 600 mg was shown to be significantly more useful compared to IM 75 mg, as can be seen in table VI. In the TA group, the drug was rated very useful in 20% of the cases, and useful or very useful in 70%. The corresponding values for the IM group were 8 and 42%, respectively.

Discussion

Based on this comparative double-blind study it is evident that TA given 600 mg daily in three divided doses is highly effective in relieving symptoms of osteoarthritis of the knee. Furthermore, one can expect superior efficacy, safety, patient toleration and usefulness in comparison to IM in a usual daily dosage of 75 mg. In Japan, IM is most commonly used in a dose of 25 mg given three times daily. For many years, IM has been widely used throughout the world for the treatment of various inflammatory and painful disorders of the locomotor system. As such it has come to be regarded as a standard nonsteroidal anti-inflammatory drug of proven efficacy. Since chronic pain is a major symptom of osteoarthritis of the knee, a potent analgesic activity of TA may contribute to the outstanding clinical efficacy observed in this study. In fact, TA was significantly superior to IM in the improvement rating for pain at rest, tenderness and difficulty in daily activities considered to be mainly due to pain in the knee. These activities include climbing, getting down stairs and squatting.

TA appeared to be a drug with a reasonably high degree of safety as one of the nonsteroidal anti-inflammatory agents used within a limited dosage level and duration of administration, as employed in this study. The occurrence of side effects, mostly gastrointestinal symptoms, was significantly less frequent in the TA-treated patients than those in the IM group. Given superior efficacy and safety, TA was shown to be significantly more useful as compared to IM. Based on our experience, we expect TA to be a valuable addition in the treatment of osteoarthritis of the knee.

References

1   Fujimura, H.; Tsurumi, K.; Hiramatsu, Y.; Tamura, Y.; Kuniba, S.; Yanagihara, M.:
     Pharmacological study on 5-benzoyl-α-methyl-2-thiophene acetic acid. 1. Anti-inflammatory and analgesic activity. Pharmacometrics 9: 715–725 (1975).
2   Fujimura, H.; Hiramatsu, Y.; Tamura, Y.; Maekawa, K.: Irritative action of RU 15.060

on gastromucous membrane by repeated oral administration in rats (unpublished results).

3   Nakagawa, T.; Yasuhara, T.; Hanamura, H.; Kajino, G.; Iwata, K.; Ida, K.; Mimatsu, K.; Higuchi, Y.; Sakakibara, T.; Suzuki, H.; Tagawa, N.; Umezawa, K.; Sugiura, M.; Furukawa, T.; Chiba, H.; Ohtani, N.; Sugiura, K.; Maeda, H.; Aoki, M.; Nakagawa, M.; Ito, K.; Mizuno, H.; Yokota, S.; Mabuchi, N.; Kawashima, K.: Clinical evaluation concerning the effect of tiaprofenic acid on low back pain. Jap. Pharmacol. Ther. *8:* 2807–2818 (1980).

4   Aoki, T.; Kazui, H.; Inoue, Y.; Suzuki, K.; Nagano, M.; Shibakuki, S.; Kawakami, K.; Kawaji, W.; Ohta, N.; Miyoshi, K.; Shigematsu, Y.; Abe, M.; Hayashi, M.; Shiomi, T.; Kudo, T.: Clinical study on the effect of tiaprofenic acid on neck-shoulder-arm syndrome. Jap. J. clin. exp. Med. (to be published, 1981).

5   Taguchi, T.; Fujita, M.; Hamanaka, Y.; Sakai, K.; Yamada, T.; Ashimura, M.; Kimura, S.; Tomita, K.: Clinical evaluation concerning the effect of tiaprofenic acid on post-operative pain. Jap. Pharmacol. Ther. *8:* 2761–2768 (1980).

6   Kamiya, K.; Mori, M.; Suzuki, M.; Chikada, A.: Clinical evaluation concerning the effect on post-traumatic pain and inflammation, by double-blind group comparison methods between tiaprofenic acid and ibuprofen. Clin. Rep. *14:* 1619–1624 (1980).

7   Shimomura, Y.; Shinmei, M.; Ohtani, K.; Miyamoto, K.: Clinical evaluation concerning the effect of tiaprofenic acid on post-traumatic pain and inflammation. Jap. Pharmacol. Ther. *8:* 2769–2776 (1980).

8   Kageyama, T.; Yoshizawa, H.; Morinaga, T.; Warabi, H.; Aoki, T.; Fujimori, I.; Sugano, T.; Fujitsuka, M.; Koshiishi, Y.; Sato, T.; Yoshino, S.; Fukui, K.; Sugawara, S.: Results of preliminary clinical trial concerning the effect of tiaprofenic acid on chronic rheumatoid arthritis. Jap. Pharmacol. Ther. *8:* 2275–2290 (1980).

T. Kageyama, MD, Department of Orthopedic Surgery, Rheumatism and Allergy Center, Sagamihara National Hospital, Sagamihara, Kanagawa (Japan)

Rheumatology, vol. 7, pp. 173–181 (Karger, Basel 1982)

Double-Blind Comparison of a
New Anti-Inflammatory Nonsteroidal Agent,
Tiaprofenic Acid versus Sulindac in
Osteoarthritis of the Knees

A.J. Fellet, A.H. Toledo, A.S. Scotton

Service of Rheumatology, Faculty of Medicine, Federal University, Juiz de Fora, Brazil

Introduction

Research of new nonsteroidal anti-inflammatory agents is justified because of the importance of the symptomatology caused by various rheumatic illnesses and because of the often held opinion that the therapeutic activity of these drugs is inversely proportional to their tolerance.

Propionic acid derivatives, among them tiaprofenic acid [*Clemence* et al., 1974], have constituted the main group of compounds studied, having therapeutic functions which are very close to those of corticosteroids, without their frequent and severe side effects [*Lechat and Lacier,* 1975].

Tiaprofenic acid (α(5-benzoyl-2-thienyl)-propionic acid) has been reported to be a potent nonsteroidal anti-inflammatory and non-narcotic analgesic drug [*Pottier* et al., 1977].

Sulindac is an indene derivative of indomethacin [*Van Arman* et al., 1976] which has been claimed to be effective in a proportion of patients suffering from chronic rheumatic diseases and therefore seemed to be an appropriate comparative agent for a new analgesic/anti-inflammatory drug [*Bordier and Kuntz,* 1978].

The present study compared the therapeutic effect and tolerance of tiaprofenic acid with those of sulindac in patients with osteoarthritis of the knees.

Patients and Methods

We conducted a double-blind controlled clinical study in 53 adult out-patients of either sex all suffering from osteoarthritis of the knees.

Table I. Characteristics of the patients participating in the trial

Data	Tiaprofenic acid	Sulindac
Number of patients	27	26
Males	5	5
Females	22	21
Age, years		
Mean ± SD	58.56 ± 10.60	58.12 ± 9.26
Under 49	4	4
50–59	9	13
60–69	11	6
70 and over	3	3
Weight, kg		
Mean ± SD	75.19 ± 8.94	74.23 ± 10.66
Up to 59	1	1
60–69	5	8
70–79	12	10
80 and over	9	7
Duration of illness		
Mean, years; months	7; 5	4; 11
Duration of the crises		
Mean, days before the study	32	23

The following patients were excluded from the study: simultaneous involvement of the knees and hips; bone and cartilage lesions with X-ray changes corresponding to the third and fourth stages of Steinbrocker's classification; patients being treated with other nonsteroidal anti-inflammatory drugs, hypnotics or corticoids; patients undergoing physical therapy which could influence the course of their illness; patients with gastric symptomatology, peptic ulceration, recent episodes of haematemesis and those having undergone surgery; patients who were known to be allergic to aspirin or any other nonsteroidal anti-inflammatory drug; pregnant women.

The patients were randomly assigned to one of two homogeneous and parallel groups.

Tiaprofenic acid group. This group consisted of 27 patients taking tiaprofenic acid in a dosage of 600 mg per day (200 mg three times a day).

Sulindac group. Consisting of 26 patients taking sulindac in a dosage of 450 mg per day (150 mg three times a day).

Demographic data for the 2 groups is shown in table I.

In both groups, the medications were presented in capsule form of identical shape of size and patients were instructed to take one capsule three times a day with food.

Treatment was preceeded by a wash-out period of one week and the treatment in both groups was of two weeks duration. All other anti-inflammatory and analgesic treatment was stopped at the beginning of the wash-out period.

The tiaprofenic acid group had an average duration of illness of 7 years 5 months. The present crisis had begun, on average, 32 days previously (table I). These patients had previously

Table II. Previous treatments

	Tiaprofenic acid	Sulindac
No previous treatment	6	7
Previous treatment	21	19
Drug used[1]		
Nonsteroidal anti-inflammatory	12	17
Analgesics	9	8
Others	4	2

[1] Some patients received more than one other drug.

taken various medications and 81.4% of them had used anti-inflammatory and analgesic drugs (table II).

The duration of illness in the sulindac group was, on average, 4 years 11 months and their present crisis was of an average duration of 23 days. The patients in this group had also been taking various types of medication, 92.6% having taken analgesic and anti-inflammatory drugs.

Intolerance to previous drug treatment was common in both groups without there being any significant differences between them. One-way analysis of variance (Anova) between groups in relation to intolerance was not significant. The 2 treatment groups were therefore considered homogenous.

Patients admitted to the study were assessed one day before drug administration (0 day) and subsequently on the 7th and 14th days of treatment, by the same independent observer, and at the same time of the day for each patient.

Laboratory investigations including a full blood count, erythrocyte sedimentation rate (ESR), standard liver function tests, urinanalysis, blood urea and creatinine, measurement of plasma proteins and electrolytes were undertaken before and after the treatment period.

Clinical assessment was achieved by recording the severity of the following parameters on a scale 0 to 4 (nil, slight, moderate, severe, very severe):

1. Spontaneous diurnal pain
2. Spontaneous nocturnal pain
3. Pain on passive movement
4. Pain on active movement
5. Morning pain on awakening
6. Functional limitations (patient assessment)
7. Functional limitations (physician assessment)
8. Impairment of joint mobility
9. Sleep disturbance
10. Local inflammatory signs
11. Stiffness after rest

The following measures of therapeutic efficacy were used: (a) articular index score based on pain, stiffness and tenderness; (b) pain score (parameters 1 to 4 listed above); (c) side effects (intensity and relation to the drug); (d) clinical global impression of efficacy and tolerance graded from 0 to 4 (nil, poor, moderate, good, very good).

Comparison of successive clinical assessments was made by one-way analysis variance (Anova) of the scores for each product with respect to:

Articular index and pain level. The sum of scores for each patient in each treatment group at each assessment.

Table III. Mean values of clinical measurements of therapeutic efficacy

Data	Tiaprofenic acid	Sulindac	P value (Anova)
Articular index			
Days 0	24.81	22.96	NS
7	16.48	19.73	NS
14	10.19	17.50	< 0.001
Percentage of improvement			
Days 7	34	15	< 0.01
14	58	19	< 0.001
Pain level			
Days 0	12.15	11.92	NS
7	8.19	10.19	0.03
14	4.96	8.65	< 0.001
Percentage of improvement			
Days 7	32	17	0.01
14	56	25	< 0.001

The percentage of improvement. Calculated from the difference between the initial score and scores at the 7th and 14th day assessments respectively divided by the initial score.

The statistical differences existing between the 2 groups in respect of the scores of pain level, articular index and percentage improvement were tested using the one-way analysis of variance. The frequency of side effects and the clinical global impression of efficacy and tolerance were tested by the X^2 method.

Results

Group mean values of clinical efficacy are shown in table III.

Articular Index

The articular index of the tiaprofenic acid group was 24.81 ($\pm$ 6.34) on day 0 and 10.9 ($\pm$ 4.52) on the 14th day. In the sulindac group, articular index war 22.96 ($\pm$ 7.60) on day 0 and 17.50 ($\pm$ 6.86) on the 14th day. The difference between the observed indices of the two products at the last assessment showed statistical significance ($p < 0.01$) (fig. 1). The percentage improvement of articular index in the tiaprofenic acid group was 34% at the end of the 1st week and 58% at the end of the second week. The sulindac group showed a percentage improvement of articular index of 15% and 19% at the end of the first and second week respectively. The difference between the two groups at the end of the study was significant ($p < 0.01$) (fig. 2).

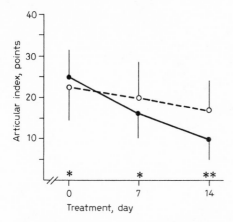

Fig. 1. Articular index at the initial assessment and on days 7 and 14 of treatment.
—— = Tiaprofenic acid; — — — = sulindac. *p = NS; **p < 0.01.

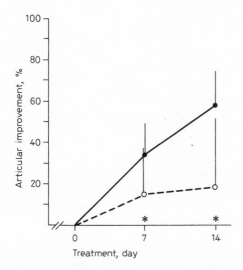

Fig. 2. Percentage of articular improvement obtained on the days 7 and 14 of treatment.
—— = Tiaprofenic acid; — — — = sulindac. *p < 0.01.

Pain Level

The initial pain level in the tiaprofenic acid group was 12.15 falling to
8.19 after 7 days treatment and to 4.96 at the end of the trial. The sulindac
group showed pain levels of 11.92 at the initial assessment and 10.19 and 8.65
at the end of the first and second weeks of treatment respectively (fig. 3).

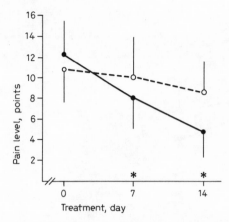

Fig. 3. Pain level at the initial assessment and on days 7 and 14 of treatment. ——— = Tiaprofenic acid; – – – = sulindac. *p < 0.01.

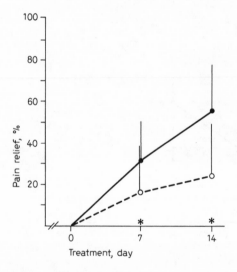

Fig. 4. Percentage of pain relief obtained on days 7 and 14 of treatment. ——— = Tiaprofenic acid; – – – = sulindac. *p < 0.01.

Statistical differences were found on the 7th day of treatment with 32% improvement in the tiaprofenic acid group and 17% improvement in the sulindac group (p = 0.01). The difference between the two groups at the 14th day of treatment was statistically significant (p < 0.001) showing 56% improvement due to tiaprofenic acid and 25% due to sulindac (fig. 4).

Table IV. Clinical Global impression after both treatments

Data	Tiaprofenic acid	Sulindac	P value (χ^2 test)
Efficiency			
A little worse or about the same	3	17	
A little better or much better	24	9	0.0005

Table V. Clinician's and patients' spontaneous reports of side-effects during trial

Data	Tiaprofenic acid Group	Sulindac	p value (χ^2 test)
Number of patients with complaints	13	18	NS
Number of complaints	14	32	
Epigastric pains	1	1	
Nausea	3	3	
Vomit	1	3	
Heartburn	4	5	
Constipation	1		
Flatulence		1	
Diarrhea		2	
Dizziness	1	5	
Insomnia		3	
Pruritus	1	3	
Headache	2	5	
Edema		1	

Clinical Global Impression

The clinical global impression of efficacy at the end of treatment (table IV) showed an improvement of the symptomatology in 24 (88.9%) of the 27 patients in the tiaprofenic acid group and 9 (34.6%) of the 26 patients in the sulindac group. This difference between the two experimental groups was statistically significant ($p < 0.01$).

Clinical Tolerance

Gastrointestinal complaints such as heartburn and epigastric pain occurred in both of the treatment groups (table V). Ten of the complaints came from the tiaprofenic acid group and 15 from the sulindac group. Other complaints were not related to the tested products. Statistical analysis of side effects between groups shows no significant differences. In general terms, biological tolerance was excellent in both groups. All laboratory values both before and after treatment were within normal limits.

Discussion

The present study compared tiaprofenic acid in a dosage of 600 mg per day with sulindac in a dosage of 450 mg per day.

Our results show that tiaprofenic acid has analgesic and anti-inflammatory activity superior to sulindac. A particularly significant difference was noted in the relief of pain, which is especially distressing and restricitve to patients with osteoarthritis of the knee.

The analgesic effect is in conformity with the results previously reported by *Cutting and Thornton* [1981] which showed superior activity of tiaprofenic acid 200 mg three times a day in comparison with aspirin 600 mg three times a day in pain following injury.

Our results showing the analgesic effects of tiaprofenic acid compliment those of *Daymond* et al. [1979] who demonstrated the superiority of tiaprofenic acid (200 mg three times a day) over ibuprofen (400 mg three times a day) as an anti-inflammatory agent in the treatment of rheumatoid arthritis.

An important consideration in the evaluation of a new drug for the treatment of osteoarthritis is the incidence of side effects. In the present study, both drugs were well tolerated, side effects being of little importance in either group and it was not necessary to interupt treatment because of them. These findings confirm the results previously reported by *Bordier and Kuntz* [1978] for sulindac and by *Peyron and Chigot* [1977] for tiaprofenic acid.

Laboratory values in this and in previously reported studies have not shown significant change due to tiaprofenic acid. The slight changes previously reported with sulindac by *Chahade and Josef* [1978] were not detected by us.

In conclusion, the present study has shown that the analgesic and anti-inflammatory activity of tiaprofenic acid is significantly superior to sulindac whilst tolerance was comparable for both drugs.

These results clearly indicate that tiaprofenic acid is useful in the clinical treatment of osteoarthritis of the knees.

Acknowledgements

Tiaprofenic acid (Surgam) tablets were supplied by Sarsa Laboratories (Roussel-Brazil). We are grateful to Dr. *H. Rodrigues* and Dr. *S. Warman* for statistical analysis.

References

Bordier, Ph.; Kuntz, D.: Sulindac: clinical results of treatment of osteoarthritis. Eur. J. Rheumatol. Inflamm. *1:* 27–30 (1978).

Camp, A.: Tiaprofenic acid in the treatment of rheumatoid arthritis. Rheumatol. Rehabil. *20:* 181–183 (1981).

Chahade, W.H.; Josef, H.: Clinical evaluation of efficacy and tolerance of Sulindac in patients with osteoarthritis of the hip and/or knee during 144 weeks: comparative study with aspirin during the first 96 weeks. Eur. J. Rheumatol. Inflamm. *1:* 41–44 (1978).

Clemence, F.; Le Martret, O.; Fournex, R.; Plassard, G.; Dagnaux, M.: Recherche de composés anti-inflammatoires et analgésiques dans la série du tiophène. Eur. J. med. Chem., Chim. ther. *9:* 390–396 (1974).

Cutting, C.J.; Thornton, E.J.: Comparative trial of tiaprofenic acid (Surgam) versus aspirin in the control of pain following injury. Pharmacol. Ther. *2:* 509–512 (1981).

Daymond, T.J.; Thompson, M.; Akbar, F.A.; Chestnet, V.: A controlled trial of tiaprofenic acid versus ibuprofen in rheumatoid arthritis. Rheumatol. Rehabil. *18:* 257–260 (1979).

Deraedt, R.; Jonguey, S.; Delevallee, F.; Flahant, M.: Release of prostaglandins E and F in an algogenic reaction and its inhibition. Eur. J. Pharmacol. *61:* 17–24 (1980).

Katona, S.G.; Burgos Vargas, R.: Acido tiaprofenico en el tratamiento de osteoarthritis. Inv. Med. Int. *7:* 86–91 (1980).

Lechat, P.; Lagier, G.: Mécanismes pharmacologiques des effets indésirables des corticoïdes. Cordicoïdes R.P. *25:* 1103–1109 (1975).

Ochoa, J.V.; Chávez, V.: Estudio clinico comparativo del acido tiaprofénico vs. indometacina en la gonartrosis. Compendium *1:* 46–57 (1980).

Peyron, J.; Chigot, D.: Etude statistique d'essais comparatifs à double insu d'un nouvel anti-inflammatoire: l'acide tiaprofénique. Med. Afr. Noire *24:* 249–252 (1977).

Pottier, J.; Berlin, D.; Raynaud, J.P.: Pharmacokinetics of the anti-inflammatory tiaprofenic acid in humans, mice, rabbits and dogs. J. pharm. Sci. *66:* 1030–1036 (1977).

Sebastian, O.; Torres, D.; Dorti, I.N.: Estudio comparativo double ciego de la actividad del acido tiaprofénico y la fenilbutazona en el tratamiento de las gonartrosis. Prensa méd. argent. *66:* 375–379 (1979).

Valdes, E.F.: Estudio de la accion del acido tiaprofénico en la artritis gotosa aguda por comparacion con la fenilbutazona. Semana méd., B. Aires *155:* 127–133 (1979).

Van Arman, C.G.; et al.: Pharmacology of Sulindac; in Huskisson, Franchimont, Clinoril in the treatment of rheumatic disorders (Raven Press, New York 1976).

Van Eslande, Ph.: Etude comparative en double-aveugle de l'acide tiaprofénique et de l'indométacine dans les traitements des coxarthroses. Ars Med., Brux. *35:* 1393–1402 (1980).

Wojtulwski, J.; Walter, J.; Thornton, E.J.: Tiaprofenic acid (Surgam) in the treatment of osteoarthritis of the knee and hip. Rheumatol. Rehabil. *20:* 177–180 (1981).

A. Fellet, MD, Department of Rheumatology, Faculty of Medicine,
Rua do Sampaio 375, 36100 Juiz de Fora, MG (Brazil)

Rheumatology, vol. 7, pp. 182–187 (Karger, Basel 1982)

Evaluation of Surgam: Long-Term Tolerance

J. Meurice

'Le Valdor' Gerontological Centre, Liège, Belgium

Introduction

A sad characteristic of degenerative rheumatism is its persistence. It thus requires frequent and often long treatment with analgesic and anti-inflammatory agents. Unfortunately, all too frequently one hears that a rheumatic patient treated his rheumatism for 6 months and then his stomach for a further 6 months. This was related to the ingestion of old, nonsteroid antiinflammatory agents. The new generation has sought to improve this situation and the present study was aimed at demonstrating the long-term tolerance of Surgam in patients suffering from osteoarthrosis.

Method

Treatment. Patients were treated for 60–62 weeks with 600 mg of Surgam in three divided doses per day. No other antiinflammatory or analgesic agent was accepted. By contrast, treatment by physiotherapy was allowed.

Patients. 30 hospitalized patients of both sexes suffering from osteoarthrosis ot the hip or knee were included in the trial. Excluded from the trial were those with a past history of hematemesis from peptic ulcer, gastric discomfort or disease, treatment with anticoagulants, pregnancy, etc. The study was undertaken on an open basis.

Evaluation. The patients were evaluated monthly. The principal aim of the trial being to study the patients' tolerance of the substance, it was felt to be also opportune to evaluate, at the same time, its long-term efficacy. Efficacy was scored monthly as excellent, very good, good, satisfactory poor. Tolerance was assessed monthly on the basis of: (1) spontaneous complaints by the patients; (2) hematological examinations: hemoglobin, hematocrit, red cell count, white cell count, platelets, differential white cell count, ESR, corpuscular value; (3) biochemical examinations: alkaline phosphatase, creatinine, serum iron, fibrinogen, protein, cholesterol, esterified cholesterol, triglycerides, SGOT, SGPT, LDH, glucose, urea, lipids, and electrolytes; (4) urine: protein, glucose, microscopy.

Table I. Details of patients and duration of tiaprofenic acid treatment

Patient No.	Age on entry, years	Sex	Weight on entry, kg	Date of entry	Date of last assessment	Number of weeks in trial
1	74	F	79	26. 4. 74	27. 6. 75	60
2	71	M	84	26. 4. 74	27. 6. 75	60
3	81	F	69	30. 7. 74	26. 9. 75	60
4	71	F	63	19. 9. 74	28. 11. 75	61
5	73	M	58	15. 10. 74	26. 12. 75	62
6	81	F	83	4. 11. 74	19. 1. 76	62
7	68	M	91	4. 11. 74	19. 1. 76	62
8	72	F	75	13. 1. 75	1. 4. 76	62
9	81	F	52	21. 1. 75	26. 3. 76	60
10	52	F	81	10. 3. 75	19. 5. 76	61
11	79	M	78	10. 3. 75	19. 5. 76	61
12	74	F	58	30. 5. 75	30. 7. 76	60
13	78	F	72	8. 9. 75	18. 11. 76	61
14	58	F	92	8. 9. 75	18. 11. 76	61
15	73	F	89	8. 9. 75	18. 11. 76	61
16	77	M	55	28. 10. 75	31. 12. 76	60
17	68	M	92	12. 1. 76	28. 3. 77	62
18	74	F	67	12. 1. 76	28. 3. 77	62
19	77	F	83	12. 1. 76	28. 3. 77	62
20	69	F	72	21. 1. 76	25. 3. 77	60
21	82	F	50	9. 4. 76	2. 6. 77	59
22	64	M	57	13. 4. 76	17. 6. 77	60
23	79	M	74	4. 5. 76	15. 7. 77	62
24	72	F	69	26. 5. 76	29. 7. 77	60
25	69	M	88	1. 7. 76	9. 9. 77	61
26	70	F	68	6. 9. 76	21. 11. 77	62
27	74	F	63	6. 9. 76	21. 11. 77	62
28	81	M	65	28. 9. 76	2. 12. 77	60
29	64	M	78	2. 5. 77	3. 7. 78	60
30	57	F	62	6. 9. 77	6. 11. 78	60

Results

Patients. 30 patients participated in the study which lasted for a period of 60–62 weeks. The age range was 57–82 years. There were 11 men and 19 women. Data are shown in table I. Joint disorders and other pathology are summarized in table II.

Table II. Osteoarthritis and concomitant diseases

Patient No.	Osteoarthritis	Concomitant diseases
1	Hip	diabetes, cardiomyopathy
2	Hip	none
3	Hip	diabetes, Paget's disease,
4	Hip	bronchial emphysema
5	Hip	prostatism,
6	Knees	cholelithiasis, obesity
7	Knee	degenerative cervical spine disease
8	Knees	none
9	Hip	left ventricular hypertrophy, arterial hypertension, Paget's disease
10	Knee	obesity
11	Knees	sciatica, endarteritis, angina, hyperlipidemia
12	Hip	none
13	Knees	angina, osteomalacia,
14	Knees	degenerative cervical spine disease, bronchitis, insomnia
15	Knee	arterial hypertension, angina, obesity
16	Hip	chronic bronchitis,
17	Knee	chronic bronchitis
18	Knee	spastic colon, hemorrhoids, Paget's disease
19	Knee	diabetes, hyperlipidemia, obesity,
20	Hip	arrhythmia, angina,
21	Hips	cardiopathy
22	Hip	asthma
23	Hip	diabetes, chronic bronchitis
24	Hip	asthma, diverticular disease
25	Hip	anthracosilicosis, prostatism
26	Knee	none
27	Knee	rheumatoid arthritis, varicose ulcers,
28	Hips	chronic bronchitis, prostatism
29	Knees	none
30	Knee	gastritis, arterial hypertension

Efficacy. Evaluation of efficacy as scored by the team is summarized in table III, being either satisfactory or good, with a majority of good.

Tolerance. Complaints of the patients are summarized in table IV. The majority of complaints were related to the digestive tract, and, to a lesser extent, involved the CNS. There were no withdrawals from the trial.

Table III. Investigator's assessment of therapeutic activity (number of patients)

	Month of trial													
	1	2	3	4	5	6	7	8	9	10	11	12	13	14
Excellent	1	1	1	1	0	0	0	0	0	0	0	0	0	0
Very good	2	3	0	0	1	1	1	1	0	1	1	1	1	1
Good	21	23	27	25	23	17	19	17	25	25	18	16	18	18
Satisfactory	5	3	2	4	5	11	9	10	4	4	10	11	9	9
Poor	1	0	0	0	0	0	0	1	0	0	1	2	2	2
Not assessed	0	0	0	0	1	1	1	1	1	0	0	0	0	0

Laboratory. A total of 34 parameters (hematology, serum biochemistry and urine) were monitored in all patients on entry into the trial, at 14-day intervals during the first three months, and afterwards at monthly-interval. As expected, there were isolated results outside normal limits both before and during the trial. However, no consistent trends were evident in mean values or in the number of patients above or below the normal ranges.

Discussion

30 patients participated in this study. Patients were selected not only on the basis of their joint condition, but also of their aptitude for participation in a long-term tolerance study. This was facilitated by the existence in our hospital of 500 'chronic hospitalization' beds. Only patients were included (1) whose tolerance to drugs was generally good; (2) patients who desired to be treated and were perfectly conscious of their role as control subjects; and (3) individuals whose life expectancy reasonably exceeded the predicted duration of the study. These criteria explain, on the one hand, the long period over which the study took place (1974–1978) and, on the other hand, the fact that there were no instances of the trial being abandoned.

Efficacy was good for the great majority of patients. Where tolerance is concerned, at first sight 23 patients presented miscellaneous complaints during the course of the trial, but these were, of course, complaints and not necessarily side effects. It is even astonishing that in this type of population and for a period of more than 1 year, there were complaints in only 23 patients. The following must be eliminated from these 23 patients: 3 patients in whom

Table IV. Individual complaints

Patient No.	Complaint	Duration	Frequency	Present before trial
1	Nausea	few days	5 times	no
	Diarrhea	persistent	persistent	yes
2	None	–	–	–
3	Heartburn	7 days	3 times	no
		15 days	once	no
	Diarrhea	daily	frequent	yes
4	Abdominal discomfort	10 days	twice	no
5	Vertigo	1 week	once	no
6	Dyspepsia	few days	4 times	no
7	Vertigo	1 week	once	no
8	Heartburn	few days	3 times	no
9	None	–	–	–
10	Heartburn	2 weeks	once	no
		few days	twice	no
	Abdominal discomfort	few days	twice	no
11	None	–	–	–
12	Heartburn	almost continuously	–	yes
13	Gastric heaviness	1 week	once	no
	Heartburn	few days	3 times	no
14	Diarrhea	habitual	–	yes
15	Nausea	few days	twice	no
16	Abdominal discomfort	few days	twice	no
17	Vertigo	few days	twice	no
18	Colitis	several days	twice	no
19	Heartburn	several days	twice	no
	Loose stools	several days	twice	no
20	None	–	–	–
21	None	–	–	–
22	Nausea	few days	3 times	no
	Heartburn	several days	once	no
23	Nausea	several days	3 times	no
	Abdominal discomfort	few days	once	no
24	Nausea	several days	once	no
	Abdominal discomfort	2 weeks	once	no
25	Nausea	several days	twice	no
	Headache	few days	once	no
26	None	–	–	–
27	None	–	–	–
28	Erythema	1–2 days	once	no
29	Abdominal discomfort	few days	once	no
30	Heartburn	several days	twice	no

diarrhea was preexistent and was related to biguanides (patients No. 1, 3, 14); 1 case of heartburn secondary to hiatal hernia (patient No. 12), and 1 case of colitis (patient No. 18).

Vertigo was reported by 3 patients with a mean age of 70 years, lasting for several days. 1 patient developed transient erythema which disappeared spontaneously without any interruption in the administration of Surgam and without the prescription of an antihistamine. With regard to the other cases, even though the complaints may be imputed to the administration of the drug, their slight degree, short duration and rarity was such that they may be considered as being negligible in a period of continuous treatment of 14 months. It is also important to bear in mind the psychological aspect in such patients who, at any given time, could have rejected such long-term therapy as a result of such complaints. Laboratory investigations revealed no notable changes.

Conclusions

Tiaprofenic acid studied in a geriatric hospital context for a period of 14 months in 30 patients with major osteoarthrosis of the hip or knee proved to be well tolerated with good efficacy. Side effects were benign and nonsignificant. Hematological and biochemical tolerance was excellent. Nothing emerged in this study to suggest a contraindication to the long-term use of tiaprofenic acid.

J. Meurice, MD, Centre Gérontologique 'Le Valdor', 145 rue Basse-Wez, B-4020 Liège (Belgium)

Rheumatology, vol. 7, pp. 188–193 (Karger, Basel 1982)

Simultaneous Bioavailability of Tiaprofenic Acid (Surgam) in Serum and Synovial Fluid in Patients with Rheumatoid Arthritis

T.J. Daymond[a], R. Herbert[b]

[a]District General Hospital, and [b]Department of Pharmacy, Sunderland Polytechnic, Sunderland, England

Introduction

Tiaprofenic acid [α-(5-benzoyl-2-thienyl)-propionic acid] has been shown in animal studies to be a potent anti-inflammatory and non-narcotic analgesic [3, 5]. A dose of 200 mg t.d.s. has been shown to be effective in the treatment of rheumatoid arthritis [1, 4] and osteoarthritis [14, 15]. A pharmacokinetic study in healthy volunteers has shown that tiaprofenic acid has a half-life in plasma of only approximately 1.7 h which is independent of dose [7]. The present study was conducted to determine the serum and synovial fluid profiles of the drug in patients suffering from rheumatoid arthritis.

Patients and Methods

7 patients (1 male and 6 females) aged 46–69 years, suffering from active rheumatoid arthritis and requiring knee aspiration were studied. All patients were receiving long-term treatment with tiaprofenic acid 200 mg t.d.s. One patient was also taking glibenclamide, 10 mg daily, for diabetes mellitus.

Patients took their dose of tiaprofenic acid at 22.00 h on the evening prior to the study and fasted overnight. On the study day the usual 200 mg morning dose of tiaprofenic acid was administered at 9.00 h under supervision. Blood and synovial fluid samples were taken immediately before and throughout an 8-hour period after this study dose (fig. 1). Breakfast was taken after the second blood sample. Serum and synovial fluid samples were assayed for tiaprofenic acid by high-performance liquid chromatography [14].

Results

Typical serum and synovial fluid profiles of tiaprofenic acid are shown in figures 2–6. Absorption into the serum was rapid. Peak serum levels were

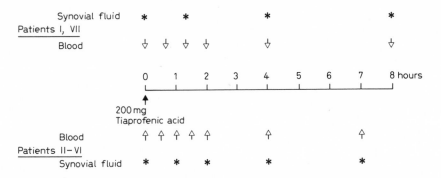

Fig. 1. Sampling times.

seen within 90 min of the study dose in all patients (table I) with a mean value of $26.0 \mu g/ml$ (table II). Serum half-lives were short with a mean value of 1.56 h.

In contrast, synovial fluid concentrations remained relatively constant throughout the 8-hour period and the profiles were independent of the serum concentration. At baseline, 11 h after the previous dose, tiaprofenic acid was detected in the synovial fluid of all patients and the mean level exceeded that in the serum (table II). In contrast to serum levels, synovial fluid levels reached approximately $5 \mu g/ml$ and remained relatively constant, exceeding serum levels after 4–6 h.

Further evidence of the independence of the synovial fluid profile is shown in patient VI (fig. 7). This patient mistakenly took an extra dose of tiaprofenic acid 1.5 h before the study dose. Synovial fluid levels were initially high in this patient and remained at $5 \mu g/ml$ over the 8 h, exceeding the serum levels over the latter half of this period.

In addition to tiaprofenic acid patient V was taking glibenclamide, 10 mg daily, for maturity onset diabetes mellitus, but showed typical serum and synovial fluid profiles (fig. 6). Patient VII mistakenly took only half the proposed dose. Serum and synovial fluid levels in this patient were correspondingly low but nevertheless showed typical profiles (fig. 8).

Discussion

This study shows that tiaprofenic acid is rapidly absorbed and eliminated from the serum and that it does not accumulate in the serum with long-term treatment in patients suffering from rheumatoid arthritis. These

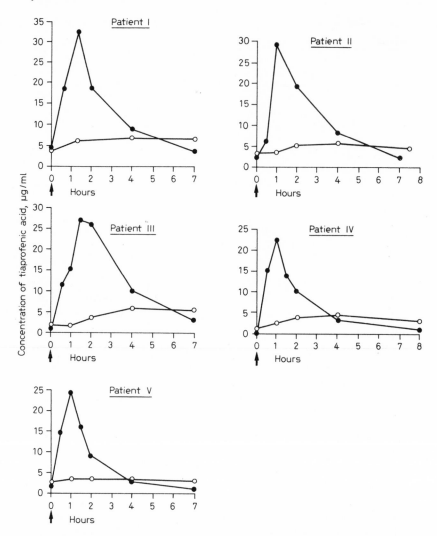

Fig. 2–6. Typical serum and synovial fluid profiles of tiaprofenic acid. ● = Serum; ○ = synovial fluid; ↑ = 200 mg tiaprofenic acid.

findings are similar to those of *Pottier* et al. [11] in studies in healthy volunteers, thus indicating that the bioavailability of the drug is not altered in rheumatoid arthritis.

Secondly it shows that tiaprofenic acid penetrates the synovial membrane and is retained at relatively constant levels within the synovial fluid.

Table I. Tiaprofenic acid in serum following 200-mg study dose in patients receiving 200 mg t.d.s.

Patient No.	Time to peak min	Half-life h
I	80	1.95
II	90	1.55
III	90	1.72
IV	60	1.44
V	60	1.52
VI	90	1.18
(VII)	(40)	(0.86)
Mean (excluding VII)	78	1.56

Patient VII took only half the proposed dose.

Table II. Concentrations of tiaprofenic acid (µg/ml) in serum and synovial fluid (SF) following 200 mg study dose in patients receiving 200 mg t.d.s.

Patient No.	0 hour		Peak		Final sample	
	serum	SF	serum	SF	serum	SF
I	4.7	3.9	32.2	6.9	3.9	6.4
II	2.0	3.1	29.6	5.9	2.0	4.3
III	1.1	1.3	27.0	6.0	3.2	5.3
IV	0.1	0.8	22.7	4.5	1.0	2.5
V	1.8	2.7	24.3	3.6	1.0	3.0
VI	5.9[a]	4.8[a]	20.5	5.1	0.7	4.6
(VII)	(zero)	(0.4)	(11.1)	(1.1)	(0.2)	(0.6)
Mean (excluding VII)	1.9	2.4	26.0	5.3	2.0	4.4

Patient VII took only half the proposed dose.
[a] Excluded from mean. See figure 7.

Synovial fluid levels of tiaprofenic acid exceeded those in the serum at baseline (11 h after the previous dose) and again during the excretion phase after 4–6h. Single dose studies of acetylsalicylic acid [12], flurbiprofen [2], indomethacin [6] and ketoprofen [10] have shown that concentrations of these drugs in synovial fluid also exceed those in serum during the excretion phase. The mechanism by which synovial fluid concentrations of tiaprofenic

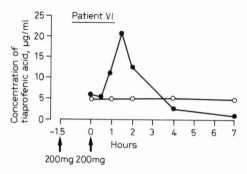

Fig. 7. Serum (●) and synovial fluid (○) profiles of tiaprofenic acid.

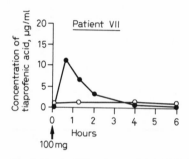

Fig. 8. Serum (●) and synovial fluid (○) profiles of tiaprofenic acid.

acid and these other non-steroidal anti-inflammatory drugs are maintained at levels exceeding those in serum remains obscure.

Tiaprofenic acid has been shown to be a potent inhibitor of prostaglandin synthetase with an IC_{50} of $0.034 \mu g/ml$ in vitro [9]. Synovial fluid levels of tiaprofenic acid in the present study exceeded this IC_{50} concentration by at least ten-fold in all samples. It is therefore interesting to speculate that tiaprofenic acid may act, at least in part, by inhibiting prostaglandin synthetase within synovial fluid.

Huskisson et al. [8] have suggested that plasma levels of non-steroidal anti-inflammatory drugs do not parallel clinical action so that drugs with short plasma half-lives can be effective given once or twice daily. Our findings suggest that this may be true of tiaprofenic acid. This possibility is currently being investigated.

Acknowledgement

We are grateful to the editor of *Rheumatology and Rehabilitation* for permission to publish this paper, and to Miss *M. Jolly* for help with this study.

References

1 Camp, A.V.: Tiaprofenic acid in the treatment of rheumatoid arthritis. Rheumatol. Rehabil. *20:* 181–183 (1981).

2 Chalmers, T.M.; Glass, R.C.; Marchant, B.: Concentrations of flurbiprofen in serum and synovial fluid from patients with active rheumatoid disease. Br. J. clin. Pract., suppl. 9, pp. 3–5 (1980).

3 Clemence, F.; Le Martret, O.; Fournex, R.; Plassard, G.; Dagnaux, M.: Recherche de composes anti-inflammatoires et analgésiques dans la série thiophene. Eur. J. med. chem. *9:* 390–396 (1974).

4 Daymond, T.J.; Thompson, M.; Akbar, F.A.; Chestney, V.: A controlled trial of tiaprofenic acid versus ibuprofen in rheumatoid arthritis. Rheumatol. Rehabil. *18:* 257–260 (1979).

5 Deraedt, R.; Jocquey, S.; Delevallee, F.; Flahaut, M.: Release of prostaglandins E and F in algogenic reaction and its inhibition. Eur. J. Pharmacol. *61:* 17–24 (1980).

6 Emori, H.W.; Champion, G.O.; Bluestone, R.; Paulus, H.E.: Simultaneous pharmacokinetics of indomethacin in serum and synovial fluid. Ann. rheum. Dis. *32:* 433–435 (1973).

7 Eve, N.O.; Jolly, M.: The relative bioavailability of different tiaprofenic formulations; unpublished report (Roussel Laboratories 1981).

8 Huskisson, E.C.; Scott, J.; Christophidis, N.: How frequently should anti-inflammatory drugs be given? A study with indoprofen. Rheumatol. Rehabil. *20:* 174–176 (1981).

9 Jocquey, S.; Deraedt, R.: Effect of tiaprofenic acid on biosynthesis of prostaglandins; unpublished report (Roussel-Uclaf AD77, 1976).

10 Mitchell, W.S.; Scott, P.; Kennedy, A.C.; Brooks, P.M.; Templeton, R.; Jeffries, M.G.: Clinico-pharmacological studies on ketoprofen ('Orudis'). Curr. med. Res. Opin. *3:* 423–430 (1975).

11 Pottier, J.; Berlin, D.; Raynaud, J.P.: Pharmacokinetics of the anti-inflammatory tiaprofenic acid in humans, mice, rats, rabbits and dogs. J. pharm. Sci. *66:* 1030–1036 (1977).

12 Sholkoff, S.D.; Eyring, E.J.; Rowland, M.; Riegelman, S.: Plasma and synovial fluid concentrations of acetylsalicylic acid in patients with rheumatoid arthritis. Arthritis Rheum. *10:* 348–351 (1967).

13 Van Eslande, P.: Comparative double-blind study of tiaprofenic acid and indomethacin in the treatment of osteoarthritis of the hip. Ars. Med., Brux. *35:* 1393–1402 (1980).

14 Ward, G.T.; Stead, J.A.; Freeman, M.: A rapid and specific method for the determination of tiaprofenic acid in human plasma. J. Liq. Chromatogr. (in press).

15 Wojtulewski, J.A.; Walter, J.; Thornton, E.J.: Tiaprofenic acid (Surgam) in the treatment of osteoarthritis of the knee and hip. Rheumatol. Rehabil. *20:* 177–180 (1981).

T.J. Daymond, MB, MRCP, Consultant in Rheumatology and Rehabilitation,
District General Hospital, Kayll Road, Sunderland SR4 7TP (England)

Rheumatology, vol. 7, pp. 194–198 (Karger, Basel 1982)

Experience with Tiaprofenic Acid (Surgam) in the Treatment of Osteoarthritis of the Hip Joint

L. Zichner

Orthopädische Universitätsklinik und Poliklinik Friedrichsheim, Frankfurt a. M., BRD

The aim of the presented study was to evaluate the efficacy and tolerance of tiaprofenic acid (TA) in the symptomatic treatment of osteoarthritis of large joints in comparison with a standard therapy with indomethacin used in our clinic.

Methods and Patients

Methods

Outpatients with painful osteoarthritis of the hip joint in the radiographic stage II were included in the study. Stage II (table I) shows moderate radiographic changes with early reduction of the joint space, small osteophytes and discrete sclerotic areas.

Patients were allocated to either of two groups according to a randomization list. One group received 200 mg of TA orally, t.i.d., the other received 50 mg of indomethacin orally, t.i.d. The dosage was kept unchanged over 3 weeks. There was no further anti-rheumatic medication. Physical examinations were performed before therapy and 1 and 3 weeks later. Documentation and scoring of the results were done according to the evaluation system of *Merle d'Aubigné,* modified by *Charnley* [1], which include: pain level, walking distance, gait, articular angle during passive motion, performing complex motions and estimation of clinical results.

Patients

Ten men (table II) and 20 women of average age of 51 years (range 32–68 years) and approximately similar heights and weights showed 37 affected hips (table III) of which 35 belonged (table IV) to stage II, 2 were radiologically classified in stage I. The etiology was mostly degenerative. There was a history of approximately 3 years of pain in both groups, on the average, with a range of 1–16 years. 11 patients of the TA group and 12 patients of the indomethacin group had received various previous treatments.

As concomitant diseases, diabetes mellitus and cardiac arrhythmias were mentioned in 2 cases, the concomitant medications in these cases were an oral antidiabetic drug and a β-blocking agent, respectively.

Table I. Radiologic classification

Stage I:	no radiographic changes
Stage II:	moderate radiographic changes with early reduction of the joint space, small osteophytes and discrete sclerotic areas
Stage III:	clearly reduced joint space; additionally to the osteophytes cystic changes are seen
Stage IV:	nearly complete or complete disappearance of joint space and deformation of joint-head

Table II. Characteristics of the patients studied

Treatment	Number of patients	Age, years		Height (range) cm	Weight (range) kg
		mean	range		
TA					
Males	4			167–173	75–80
Females	11	51.9	37–64	159–171	48–92
Indomethacin					
Males	6			163–172	59–78
Females	9	49.9	32–68	156–166	51–65

Table III. Incidence of osteoarthritis of the hip

Treatment	Site of affection			Number of hips affected
	right hip	left hip	bilateral	
TA	7	4	4	19
Indomethacin	4	8	3	18

Table IV. Radiologic classification (37 affected hip joints)

Treatment	Number of patients	Number of radiologically classified hip joints		
		stage I	stage II	total
TA	15	1	18	19
Indomethacin	15	1	17	18
		2	35	37

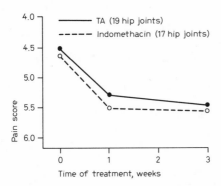

Fig. 1. Mean changes in pain level in the treatment period.

Results

No significant differences were noted between the two groups concerning age, sex, height, body weight, length of history of the disease and degree of radiographic changes. The most important parameter, the intensity of pain, which was scored (table V) from 1 to 6 points, was present at the beginning of the examination (fig. 1) in both groups to a nearly equal degree, namely 4.5 points (TA) and 4.6 points (indomethacin). The mean values of the score decreased in both groups by approximately 1 point, which means that the intensity of pain decreased equally on both treatments. Walking distance and gait changed only little in both groups. Passive joint motion was measured in degrees (table VI). Both groups initially (week 0) differed by less than 10 degrees. The improvement at the end of the treatment was about 6% in the TA group and 4% in the indomethacin group.

Table VII shows the change in passive joint motion.

The capability to perform complex motions like 'putting on stockings' or 'cutting toenails' was initially impaired in 4 patients of the TA group and in 3 patients of the indomethacin group. In the TA group, impairment of complex movements (putting on stockings) disappeared in 3 cases and for complex motion (cutting toenails), in 2 cases.

In the indomethacin group, the impairment of complex motion (putting on stockings) disappeared in 1 case.

The patients' assessment (table VIII) of the results of the treatment and that by the physician showed a comparable tendency. Both drugs, in general, were estimated to be of good efficacy.

Routine laboratory examinations showed no changes in either group.

Table V. Rating Scale for pain

1. Severe and permanent pain, even at night
2. Intensive pain, severe limitation of activity
3. Intensive but tolerable pain, limited activity
4. Mild pain during walking, no pain while resting
5. Sometimes mild pain without limitation of activity
6. No pain

Table VI. Changes in passive joint motion. Arithmetic mean and median of joint angles and their changes

Treatment	Arithmetic mean, degrees		Δ, %	Median, degrees		Δ, %
	week 0	week 3		week 0	week 3	
TA (n = 19 joints)	164.2	173.7	+ 5.8	150	165	+ 10
Indomethacin (n = 18 joints)	172.3	179.2	+ 4.0	167.5	175	+ 4.5

Table VII. Changes in passive joint motion. Assessment by score (1–6)

Treatment	Before treatment			After 3 weeks of treatment		
	IV	V	VI	IV	V	VI
TA	10	9	0	8	10	1
Indomethacin	6	10	2	5	10	3

Score: I = 0–30°; II = 31–60°; III = 61–100°; IV = 101–160°; V = 161–210°; VI = > 210°.

Table VIII. Assessment of the clinical findings

Treatment	Assessment by	Score				Number of patients
		I	II	III	IV	
TA	physician	3	12	0	0	15
	patient	5	10	0	0	15
Indomethacin	physician	6	8	1	0	15
	patient	8	7	0	0	15

Score: I = no symptoms; II = symptoms improved; III = symptoms not improved; IV = symptoms worsened.

Gastric Tolerance/Side-effects

All patients of the TA group stated a good gastric tolerance of the drug. Three patients of the indomethacin group described the gastric tolerance as moderate, the complaints were 'heartburn' in 2 cases, 'belching' and 'gastric complaints' in 1 case. Gastro-intestinal side-effects were not reported by patients of the TA group.

In the indomethacin group, transient CNS side-effects were reported in 6 cases; all 6 patients stating vertigo, in 3 patients together with dizziness and in 1 together with nausea.

Conclusion

In general, the results concerning the treatment of osteoarthritis of large joints with either TA or I are similar. The onset of the analgesic effect of I seems to start earlier.

A most important fact in view of a long term treatment seems to be, that all side-effects occured in the I-group.

Therefore, in conclusion, TA is a drug with almost the same efficacy as I, with the advantage of a better general and gastric tolerance.

Reference

Charnley, J.: The numerical grading of hips. Int. Publ. Wrightington No 20 (1968).

L. Zichner, MD, Orthopädische Universitätsklinik und Poliklinik Friedrichsheim, Marienburgstrasse 2, D-6000 Frankfurt 71 (BRD)